Artificial Intelligence in Medicine

Artificial Intelligence in Medicine

Expert systems

M. Fieschi
Faculty of Medicine
University of Marseilles

Translated by D. Cramp
Royal Free Hospital
London

SPRINGER-SCIENCE+BUSINESS MEDIA, B.V.

Original French language edition (Intelligence Artificielle en Médecine des Systèmes experts)
© Masson, Editeur, Paris, 1984
English translation published 1990
© 1990 Springer Science+Business Media Dordrecht
Originally published by Chapman and Hall in 1990
Softcover reprint of the hardcover 1st edition 1990

Typeset in 10/12 Palatino by
Best-set Typesetter Limited, Hong Kong

ISBN 978-0-412-33000-1

British Library Cataloguing in Publication Data

Fieschi, M.
  Artificial intelligence in medicine   Expert systems.
  1. Medicine. Applications of expert systems
  I. Title
  610'.28'5633

  ISBN 978-0-412-33000-1

Library of Congress Cataloging-in-Publication Data

Fieschi, M. (Marius)
    [Intelligence artificielle en médecine des systèmes experts. English]
    Artificial intelligence in medicine: expert systems /
  M. Fieschi; translated by D. Cramp.
       p.   cm.
    Translation of: Intelligence artificielle en médecine des systèmes experts.
    Includes bibliographical references.
    ISBN 978-0-412-33000-1   ISBN 978-1-4899-3428-4 (eBook)
    DOI 10.1007/978-1-4899-3428-4
    1. Artificial intelligence—Medical applications.
  2. Expert systems (Computer science)   3. Medicine—
  Decision making—Data processing.   I. Title.
  R859.7.A78F5413   1990
  610'.285'63—dc20   89-71255
                                                              CIP

Contents

Preface

Expert systems constitute a research area which is currently expanding. This book is based largely on work undertaken for my doctoral thesis and attempts to set out in readily understood language the different methods of knowledge representation used in different systems. However, since the field for applications is enormous and touches on many disciplines (engineering science, computing, geology, medicine etc.) only those systems with medical applications are presented. The second part of this book is devoted to detailed discussion of one expert system developed in this department: SPHINX.

I wish to thank all those who have given me their support, their criticisms and suggestions: Dominique Fieschi, Michel Joubert, Geneviève Botti, Michel Roux, Jean-Louis Laurière, as well as the CNRS which supported the ATP Expert Systems Group with an individual grant.

Marius Fieschi

Foreword

This work deals with 'Expert Systems' in the realm of medicine. The phrase 'Expert System' describes an information system not only in terms of its content but also in terms of its application. As with all generic terms, it is condensed to the point where the meaning cannot be guessed from simply reading it.

It concerns systems processing knowledge and behaviour in ways close to those of a human expert. In the field of medicine this expert would be the consultant or specialist to whom a family practitioner refers a 'case' which he is unable to diagnose. The study of expert systems is a branch of computer science called artificial intelligence.

Artificial intelligence, a strange phrase in which the two words taken separately conjure up opposite meanings. Intelligence seems to us to be intimately associated with human behaviour. The idea of 'artificial', on the other hand, conjures up the idea of objects characteristically not natural but 'man-made'. To call 'artificial' a prime component of human nature seems a paradox. This term is badly chosen, particularly as the aim of artificial intelligence systems is to represent behaviour comparable to human behaviour.

To gain a better grasp of the problems involved in applying artificial intelligence in medicine, let us trace the origin of the word 'intelligence'. It is derived from the Latin 'intelligentia' which is in turn derived from the verb 'intelligere': to understand. The dictionary gives the following definition of intelligence: 'The intellect in so far as it understands, in so far as it thinks; ability to understand and to understand.'

According to Larousse, intelligence is the: 'ability to understand, to make sense. The ability to adapt to a situation, to choose according to circumstances'. Whether included under the heading 'Psychology' or 'Logic' in text books of philosophy, several established ideas concerning the definition and analysis of intelligence are to be found. Most authors attribute several properties to intelligence: knowledge, understanding, memory.

Certain authors have adopted a point of view which is of particular interest to us; namely, the ability to grasp ideas which do not depend on experience. This suggests the existence of a process of reasoning which is independent of knowledge and leads to other complex processes like abstraction (conceptualization of observed facts) and generalization (finding a shape or properties common to several concepts) to achieve a more general idea.

The early accomplishments of expert systems (information systems showing intelligent behaviour and containing large quantities of human knowledge, often elicited) have shown the difference between knowledge and reasoning, a distinction barely considered by philosophers.

From this new perspective, knowledge comprises:

1. Elementary facts (or those considered as such). This is the establishment of the existence of specific facts: cough, the blood glucose level, the existence of a geological stratum, a word of a language.
2. The connection between basic facts which allow a complete description of the elementary facts to describe their properties and the associations between them.

To make use of this knowledge, or in other words to infer the existence of new facts or new properties, it is necessary to set up one or more practical techniques. The best known of these is the 'Modus Ponens': a classical term in mathematical logic which is met again in cognitive psychology. It is an elementary technique which if repeated very many times will lead to the desired result. The program which carries out this elementary technique is called the 'inference engine'.

Whatever the practical technique used, the introduction of expert systems compels one to formalize one's thinking and to analyse and express it more efficiently. Information thus 'enhanced' and better expressed becomes more efficient not only for information systems, but for man himself who in this way 'knows better what he knows and how he knows it.' The change in the attitude of mind of experts who work in this field is very clear-cut. The writing, the extraction of information, its clarity of expression, are indispensable steps in the production of expert systems, which thus involves a definite educational perspective and also necessitates formulation of hypotheses which would not have been envisaged in other circumstances.

Areas for application of expert systems in medicine are numerous and at the present time could include:

1. The diagnostic aid: where the system plays the role of the consultant.
2. The therapeutic aid: this area of application will be much more in demand. For proof of this one need only consider the numerous enquiries which crop up among medical practitioners, many of whom are uncertain how to prescribe appropriately for a given diag-

nosis, and how to adjust the prescription to the exact circumstances of the patient; also their need to know when the drug is contra-indicated.

3. Teaching: in order to teach a topic it is necessary to be conversant with it. An expert system teaching-aid must therefore of necessity contain a sub-system helping in diagnosis and/or therapy and should also adapt to the level of knowledge and 'intelligence' of its user.
4. Research aid: something about this has been said when indicating changes taking place amongst clinicians. These changes constitute an advance in the standard concept of research; moreover, expert systems can work out hypotheses, known or unknown. In this last case, these hypotheses become research objectives. Some actual examples have already been presented.
5. Biological and medical engineering: the 'automated' interpretation of functional examinations and physiological signals in the context of the specific circumstances of the patient.

The principal problems actually raised by the formulation and use of these systems are:

1. Knowledge representation: to adopt such structures that are not only general but also powerful and easy to use. The quality and theoretical backup of the inference engine including propositional logic is already well tried as to some extent is first-order logic.
2. The man-machine interface: in natural language, convenient to use though complex to analyse and appreciative of data processing resources.
3. The choice of certainty in reasoning and intervention of approximate reasoning. In this last case it is necessary to introduce numerical techniques or use the symbolic calculus. Reasoning by analogy using the calculus may be the 'solution' for dealing correctly with an uncertainty.

Such is the fascinating area dealt with in Dr Fieschi's book which is based on his doctoral thesis, in which he analyses the characteristics of the principal existing medical expert systems. It is, however, an advanced project because it also describes the system created and developed by the author based on first order logic. The work testifies to the vitality of the research within this area and also to the value of the author's achievement.

Artificial intelligence in medicine is going to take a very important place in the science of medical informatics.

This preface cannot be concluded without drawing attention to the ethical problems which will be posed by expert systems. The medical record can be divided into four stages: patient examination, the diagnostic workup, treatment and the follow-up. Undoubtedly expert systems are an aid to the preparation of the medical record, but they do not in themselves initiate patient examination: this examination is the most human part of the medical record.

The expert system will have a place alongside the well-thumbed textbook and the human specialist or consultant. In no way will the man be replaced by the machine. Any fears that this may be so are unfounded. But to allay these fears medical practice must change. This change will be genuinely influenced by the use of medical informatics and expert systems. It is up to doctors especially to assimilate the new methods and use them judiciously.

The doctor possesses a sufficiently keen critical sense when studying a published journal paper and it is this critical sense that will be exercised in using information systems. The systems will be used in no different way than a book, otherwise science without conscience will lead to the downfall of the profession.

The upheavals our society is experiencing towards the end of this century irresistibly conjure up Valery's saying: 'We, the civilized world, now know that we are mortal.'

Telecommunications and artificial intelligence are perhaps the means of allowing us to diminish man's isolation and the pressures which surround him; and through which may lie the chance of reprieve or revival.

Michel Roux

Professor in the Faculty of Medicine
of Marseille

Introduction

Within the framework of medical decision-making, whether concerning diagnosis, prognosis, therapy or prevention, the models used until recently were based mainly on theoretical concepts and probability or statistical techniques. Such methods are well known (those derived from Bayes' theorem particularly) and are readily represented in computer programs. Historically, this way of tackling the problem is very understandable, for 'calculation' is the most obvious function of the computer. Among the very numerous publications on the subjects cited by Wagner *et al.* (1978) are included the work of Gorry and Barnett (1968), de Dombal *et al.* (1972), Warner *et al.* (1972) and Salamon (1976). Yet it must be acknowledged, and indeed numerous experiments in cognitive psychology have confirmed (Elstein *et al.*, 1979), that the doctor does not recognize the role of reasoning and thought processes in computation. On that account, even when interesting results are produced (which occurs in some cases when relatively few independent variables operate), the clinician does not readily use such means because it is difficult for him to evaluate the quality of diagnostic results put forward, other than statistically. This is not satisfactory when it concerns treatment of a particular disease. For example, should a malignant tumour be treated medically, surgically or by radiotherapy when it is known that each of these therapies is only partially effective? Should two forms of treatment be combined? If medical treatment is undertaken, should it be stopped if the patient does not improve? How long should one wait? It can be assumed that the lack of acceptance by doctors of such systems-based decision-making aids is because they are based on models which do not correspond to the problems encountered. It must be said that occasionally there is a great temptation, when the model is intellectually seductive, to present the facts in such a way that they agree with the model rather than search for a model which better reflects reality.

Nevertheless, there are numerous diagnostic or therapeutic situations when a doctor needs help which might be provided by information systems. This may be the case, for example, when confronted by a rare disease or even a disease which presents in an unusual form: or again, if the patient presents with multiple pathology and conflicting pathological signs, the laboratory results may be erroneous, or there are conflicting therapeutic problems.

Artificial intelligence approaches provide attractive alternatives to the problems of decision-making. It is a domain where the main purpose of the investigator is to understand how an information analysis system may judge, compare and generalize the knowledge with which it is provided. It is concerned with operations whereby results can be obtained without knowing *a priori* how to tackle the problem. Clinical reasoning is concerned with questions of judgement, resolution of problems and decision-making, all forms of enquiry which have been tackled by researchers in cognitive psychology as well as in artificial intelligence. The psychologist wants to know how ideas are structured in the human mind, how they are developed and used. The workers in artificial intelligence want to know how to program a machine in such a way that it understands a human question, that it is capable of performing the tasks asked of it, that it reacts 'intelligently'. These two research pursuits are closely connected where the investigator in artificial intelligence thinks that the best way to approach the problem of constructing an intelligent machine is to understand human behaviour and create it by simulation.

For several years, researchers into decision-making aids in medicine have been committed to using AI methods and creating expert systems. These systems are able to process medical data and make simple but straightforward deductions in a way that makes their reasoning clear to the user. The artificial intelligence approach seeks to bypass certain limitations of the purely statistical methods by developing a more structured perception of how to cope with the problems of diagnosis or therapeutic management. The techniques used attempt to explain the deduction rules whereas statistical methods seek to extract them implicitly from collected data. The statistical approach is mainly numerical whilst the AI approach is by nature symbolic, though little separates some expert systems and the best numerical algorithms: they both apply expertise to the problem to be solved and are capable of reaching conclusions. Furthermore, these systems are interactive. They permit exchange of information between the user and the machine in a language which is often natural language. This is a strong argument in favour of a greater acceptability by users who are not computer experts. They can ask for justification of the diagnostic or therapeutic advice put forward by the system which provides the opportunity to start a dialogue with the machine that is adapted to each situation, rather than developing stereotyped questionnaires which are dull, clumsy and at times unsuitable.

Where the problem of decision-making is tackled from the viewpoint of the teaching aid, it must be emphasized that classical systems are shaped uniquely for the acquisition and control of data and not towards the way of using them. Indeed the computer has often been used for presenting the student with a pre-established questionnaire that tends to be inflexible and delivers pre-recorded 'canned data'; alternatively, source documents are provided to the student as if they were text-books or a data control tool which can be reconciled with correct answers. Even in simulation programs the development of the sequences is inflexible, and the possibilities for explanation are much reduced and not adapted to the individual student, because they have been recorded as program messages which do not make allowance for the level at which the student is working. In other words, they are lacking in educational value. We can therefore agree with Bonnet *et al.* (1981) that traditional programs are 'either unable to solve problems that they pose for they have only one ad hoc solution which is recorded once and for all; or, when they can resolve them it is done using algorithms that are impossible to decompose and therefore not suitable for educational purposes'. Artificial intelligence methods allow the development of programs able to make clear recommendations and also help in formalizing medical expertise. They give doctors a better understanding of their thought processes which is especially helpful for student teaching and the continuing education of the young doctor. Thus expertise is made available through a teaching program that relies as much on knowledge as on know-how.

What has been said may be summarized by quoting Gorry and Barnett (1973), who have suggested that decision-making systems must offer three qualities besides the relevance of their advice:

1. The possibility of holding and manipulating a set of symbolic concepts rather than simple numbers.
2. The capacity to communicate with the clinician in natural language.
3. The ability to explain the method of reasoning used.

From an historical point of view, the early work in artificial intelligence tried to solve general problems. Certain interesting general techniques were used (such as the breakdown of problems into more soluble sub-problems or the use of research heuristics) but these were inadequate in complex domains to attain the performance comparable to that of the clinical expert. More recent work during the last 10 years has, on the contrary, focused on using large amounts of data in specific domains; the work of Pople *et al.* (1975), Buchanan and Feigenbaum (1978), Shortliffe (1976), or Weiss *et al.* (1978) may be quoted. All these systems possess a level of expertise confined to a narrow domain (Pople's Internist is the exception) and the term 'expert system' has been adopted to refer to those systems which use large quantities of data. The term 'knowledge engineering' is used to describe the areas of AI which underlie the writing of expert systems: the program has become the interpreter of data and the general problem solver where heuristics play a large part in coping with the 'combinatorial explosion'. Five principal types of problems can be identified:

1. Knowledge representation: numerous methods of representation have been proposed to allow a use of knowledge by the program in a way similar to an expert in the domain. For example, Kulikowski developed a way of representing knowledge applied to ophthalmology for the diagnosis and treatment of long-term glaucoma, which models the disease process using the causal semantic network (CASNET). MYCIN created by Shortliffe's group is a consultation system in the domain of infectious disease, and is intended to provide advice in prescribing antibiotics therapy for general practitioners depending principally upon knowledge provided by experts in the form of production rules. This very important aspect of knowledge representation will be returned to later.
2. Knowledge acquisition: this is often a difficult task, especially if it is wished to give the system the ability to add to its knowledge base; in other words to have the ability to learn from examples or from data provided.
3. Methods of inference: These relate to the knowledge representation problems. Different methods are used to develop or to test hypotheses; here the problem assumes a special significance which involves judgement in the face of uncertainty.
4. Possibilities for explanation: this is a special feature of artificial intelligence systems. The methods of reasoning used are very often based on logical deduction, and allow the system to explain or justify its findings.
5. Problems of man-machine interface: these problems, like the preceding ones, are at the root of the acceptability of information systems by the non-computer worker.

All these various problems are considered through examples of existing systems before describing the SPHINX system and the results obtained in various diagnostic or therapy aid applications.

The first chapter presents general considerations which are characteristic of our approach to the problem: reflections on the possible cognitive aspect of a system using AI methods by observation of the doctors' behaviour during consultation on the possibilities of dialogue; and the ability of the system to formulate an approximate reasoning essential if it is to be of interest.

In the second chapter different methods and techniques available to tackle the crucial problem of knowledge representation are reviewed. These methods are illustrated by several expert systems particularly relevant to medicine.

The succeeding chapters are devoted to a description of the SPHINX system; its consultation programs, the knowledge acquisition and a detailed example of consultation before presenting the results obtained in two trials, namely, diagnosis of jaundice and as an aid to therapy in diabetes.

For clarity, summaries of theoretical aspects as well as certain technical terms have been relegated to the appendices.

PART ONE
Expert Systems in Medicine

1

Medical reasoning and artificial intelligence: general presentation of the problem

The task of medicine as currently practised consists of acquiring the relevant information from a patient and using it in the light of current knowledge to establish a diagnosis or to treat disease. Before considering therapy, the doctor generally postulates a sub-goal, an attempt to establish a diagnosis which explains the patient's data.

The strategy for seeking a solution by separating the problem into sub-goals is very important and much used in artificial intelligence in order to cope with combinations that are too complex to deal with. This process transforms an ill-defined problem such as 'What is this patient suffering from?' into a number of better defined sub-problems such as 'Is the jaundice caused by viral hepatitis?', or 'An acute malarial attack?', or 'Stone in the common bile duct?' Proceeding in this way by seeking appropriate evidence, the doctor's assumptions can be either confirmed or refuted. Alternative assumptions spring to mind either because of a particularly striking sign or by a combination of signs shown for a neurological study. The elementary form of medical reasoning is usually that of abductive reasoning. For example, from proposition 1. which states a fact:

1. 'If a patient has hepatitis then he presents with jaundice' and from proposition 2.
2. 'This patient presents with jaundice', a third proposition may be inferred.
3. 'This patient "perhaps" has hepatitis if he presents with jaundice.'

This inference forms the first step in reasoning which leads to the formulation of a hypothesis. From that point the doctor seeks to restrict the list of all possible hypotheses by discarding those which are inconsistent with the patient's condition, while searching for clinical and paraclinical signs which allow him on one hand to recognize these restrictions but at the same time to confirm the remaining hypotheses. The elaboration of these hypotheses occurs very early on in the consultation. It often starts with one or two salient facts being based on the heuristics which classify these diagnostic routes, like those expressed in Cutler's aphorisms: 'the commonest diseaes are common' and 'unusual symptoms are found more frequently in common diseases than common symptoms in unusual diseases.'

However, the traditional question 'Is medicine an art or a science?' reflects the difficulty and the diversity of factors that need to be taken into account in medical decision-making. The complexity of the problems presenting is often such that there exists no proof of the existence of a single solution. Moreover, doctors possess incomplete knowledge of the outlandish nature of the disease process or of the mode of action of some drugs; for all that, they have to make decisions in spite of these gaps in their knowledge. It is therefore the ability to make decisions in the face of uncertainty which leads one to speak of 'the art of medicine'.

The uncertainty arises, not only because of incomplete knowledge but also from the quality of the information gathered and the complexity of the situation, such as missing information, drug interactions which can affect laboratory results, the subjectivity of the doctor and patient stress.

Referring to Murphy's classification quoted by Williams (1982) there are four diagnostic approaches: the exhaustive, the Gestalt, the algorithmic and the hypothetico-deductive approaches.

The exhaustive approach cannot be recommended as a method generally applicable for routine application.

The second approach refers to Gestalt theory (the German word for form, shape) developed by German psychologists in the 1930s to offer a new explanation of psychological aspects of perception. It rejects the possibility of breaking down such phenomena into their constituent parts. In other words, it affirms that the interpretation of certain elements cannot be derived from the sum of its parts. It considers ideas of intuition and non-verbal information as, for example, when an expert instantly recognizes the appearance of a patient presenting with peritonitis (Williams, 1982) which involves feature recognition.

The algorithmic approach suggests that knowledge rules are not ambiguous and thus a guide to action may be developed in a sequential manner. These algorithms achieve a true base architecture, which allows identification of the main events as they present themselves. It seems that these two latter approaches are involved in the hypothesis formulation phase in medicine. The flow chart or, alternatively, the branching tree structure does not allow flexibility and is not able to take into account diseases which present in multiple forms, nor does it take account of the disease context; in other words, a collection of facts which ought to be considered and aggregated in order to describe the situation in which a knowledge is applicable. Such an approach lacks insight.

The hypothetico-deductive approach depends upon data acquisition itself. When the hypothesis has been formulated the necessary complimentary observations are provided either to confirm or refute the hypothesis. This approach can be used in a physio-pathological framework. However, this model is rarely complete and the problem of decision-making in the context of uncertainty has to be considered. It is not felt that these different approaches are mutually exclusive and in order to understand the problem with which the doctor is confronted a subtle mixture of the different approaches is used.

One of the basic principles which lead to an understanding of clinical reasoning is the 'limited rationality' of Newell and Simon (1972). The human capacity for reasoning is limited by our ability to cope with only a restricted number of facts at a time. In order to overcome these natural limitations recourse is made to certain strategies. Over a short period it is not possible to work efficiently with all the knowledge on a subject in our possession or with all the facts which can be gathered. A simple representation of a selection of facts, which appear to be the most important, is necessary. The view that computer processing might overcome these limitations of reasoning ability would be incorrect, for the increase in the number of hypotheses taken into account will not replace their relevance. This justifies our analytical approach to the strategies commonly used.

The widely used strategy of generation of hypotheses has already been alluded to. Many authors, including Pauker et al. (1976) and Kassirer and Gorry (1978), have shown that the clinician quickly generates a small number of hypotheses based on a very limited number of facts. Often the facts obtained in the early stages of consultation are sufficient to establish this limited list of hypotheses. Incorrect reasoning at the outset leads to a multiplicity of diagnostic hypotheses. According to Elstein et al. (1979) there are four principal components of this reasoning process:

1. Acquisition of information by questioning and during the clinical examination.
2. Generation of hypotheses: the number of 'active' hypotheses generated is usually few, normally of the order of four or five, rarely more than six or seven. Kassirer and Gorry (1978) have shown that the number of hypotheses formulated is small for the expert but is considerably greater for non-experts. This hypothesis generation develops as all aspects of the disease process are considered. They

usually spring to mind as a result of a particular salient feature or from a combination of factors. Pople (1982) affirms that in order to generate these hypotheses the clinician develops from experience an associative network which enables him to limit the number of possible alternative hypotheses. Elstein *et al.* (1979), however, considers that the physio-pathological models are not used enough in this early formulation of hypotheses and Pauker *et al.* (1976) observes that the generation of hypotheses develops with experience and that it is ultimately achieved with a good degree of reliability. Also, it is pointed out that when the process fails, for instance with medical students, a much more structured and algorithmic approach is used. But at times it is not the lack of data which is the cause of misdiagnosis, but the amount of 'know-how' which can be used. In an experiment carried out by Bordage (1980), a group of doctors were presented with details of 20 short clinical cases and were required to make a diagnosis in a set period of time. Each doctor taking part in the experiment was asked to reply to 70 questions that involved data concerning the 20 cases, by answering true or false. Bordage obtained evidence in this experiment that 40% of the cases were incorrectly diagnosed or inappropriate decisions had been made and that 5% of the answers to the questions involving pure fact were incorrect. It was concluded from the results of this experiment that pure knowledge of the cases was rarely used in reaching a decision. The classification of the hypotheses in order of their decreasing prevalence constitutes, according to Elstein (1979), the way of obtaining an optimum throughput. This is why a hypothesis of viral hepatitis will precede that of cancer of the liver in a list of causes of jaundice.

The hypotheses allow the organization of available data and thus to extend the human capacity to memorize large amounts of data; from this it is concluded that it is not possible to carry on an effective consultation without first having formulated a hypothesis or hypotheses that one then attempts to verify. This early generation of hypotheses appears to be the strategy most commonly used by the practitioner for diagnosis but does present crucial problems.

3. The signs are interpreted in the light of the hypotheses.
4. Hypothesis evaluation: the signs to be tested are grouped and weighted to find out whether a hypothesis can be confirmed. If not, the problem is reconsidered, new hypotheses are formulated and, if necessary, new data elicited. However, confirmation of a hypothesis usually occurs intuitively even though it may not be necessarily correct. How often is a diagnosis of myocardial infarction invalidated at autopsy?

The evaluation of a hypothesis is made in the light of the information available and knowledge of the pathology. This very attractive method, based on a conceptual model, needs a further necessary step to rationalize any decision. In other words the doctor may wish to understand 'what is going on'. However, the models are rarely complete and certainly many aspects of pathological mechanisms remain obscure which may leave the doctor to make decisions in spite of limited knowledge.

It is not absolutely necessary for a decision support system to imitate the expert in his reasoning steps, but it is useful for many reasons; in particular, it allows explanation in familiar medical terms. Moreover, evaluation of the system can be made by the human expert using his own behaviour as a reference. One of the criteria for judging a system is its ability to solve a case that is considered difficult and use the results to assess its performance. If the user does not understand the machine decision it is important that the system provides explanations that are in accord with his method of reasoning and his knowledge. To this extent study of our reasoning processes is very instructive and can lead to the formalization of medical expertise and thereby allow doctors to understand better what they know. Equally, in the long term it permits development of different strategies for resolving clinical problems by showing how in different circumstances some approaches may be more appropriate than others. While one is tempted to provide strategies for medical problems, these problems may be only particular cases of more general problems. This area has been much studied not only by psychologists interested in human reasoning but also by mathematicians, computer scientists and more recently by medical teachers. Among the objectives of artificial intelligence is the incorporation of these approaches into functional computer programs, and in fact development of programs has owed more to human reasoning than to pure mathematical methods. It is important then to keep up-to-date with the methods of thinking, of reasoning and the know-how of experts. It is an important contribution to the methods of artificial intelligence for these problems can rarely be resolved mathematically, no matter how sophisticated the formulae may be.

These AI methods have been used to develop medical consultation systems which present the user with expert findings in a particular domain. A key problem in the development of such systems is the representation of the knowledge used by the human expert in the domain. This difficult problem is further complicated by the fact that this knowledge is often inaccurate or ambiguous. Moreover, the intricate relationship between uncertain and explicit human reasoning is often very significant. It is also difficult to decide that if given sufficient information on a sufficient number of variables, when a probabilistic model becomes virtually, to use Szolovits terminology, a 'categorical' model. In any case the elements which describe the decision space are of necessity expressed in a 'categorical' manner (Williams, 1982).

Assessing the measure of credibility of a hypothesis or of a fact is difficult and is a source of much interest (Zadeh, 1965; Shafer, 1976; Szolovits and Pauker, 1978). However, it can be said there is not one good solution amongst any of the proposed forms of representation. The development of structures and rules of approximate inferences and their wide use in artificial intelligence present validation problems.

Imprecision resulting from the numerous sources and components have been listed by Buchanan (1981) who quotes in his list of sources of uncertainty, missing or erroneous facts, missing or erroneous rules and inaccuracy of the model. He enumerates the methods that are usually employed in expert systems to correct these uncertainties: recall of redundant facts and rules and use of expert heuristics.

It is important to emphasize the reasons for uncertainty: the first being linked with the abductive nature of clinical reasoning which tries to direct observations towards a generalized conclusion. This first component of uncertainty is associated with probabilities and their estimations. This is why numerous authors have tried to produce systems based on Bayes' theorem. It is a question of taking into account the prevalence of a disease, the frequency of a given disease in the presence of a given symptom, etc. But their probabilities may only be obtained in the case of fairly simple problems; it is not possible to provide them for complex problems. If the probability values are given by the expert and not estimated through observations of the frequency of appearance of a disease from present signs, the subjective probability then reflects only a degree of belief and not an observed frequency. This degree of belief completes the psychological process used in making the estimate. Much work has shown that human experts tend to ignore probabilistic reasoning (Tversky and Kahneman, 1974).

The second cause of uncertainty is brought about as a result of missing or incorrect data. In this category can also be included the inaccuracy associated with certain types of data that are difficult to elicit. For example, it is known that hepatomegaly is a sign which is difficult to detect; on that account the state of absence of hepatomegaly becomes an uncertain fact.

The third cause of uncertainty concerns missing rules, so there are particular situations with which the system is not able and does not know how to cope. It is recognized (Szolovits and Long, 1982) that the methodology used in artificial intelligence is useful in solving some of these problems. While other methods, statistical methods in particular, concede a limited number of erroneous conclusions as necessary consequences of their model, the AI approach assumes that the inclusion of additional data leads to system resolution. The introduction of weighted rules gives the possibility of expressing knowledge in a more synthetic, more concise form; moreover, this possibility is of particular interest when there are difficulties in making clear and categorizing the exact criteria on which a decision is based.

Is it because 'a pain is intense' or rather because 'it has a characteristic radiation' that the doctor is led to formulate a particular hypothesis? Each of these elements contributes information and it is interesting to be able to weigh the relative importance of each element.

The fourth cause of uncertainty is a result of a model which is incomplete or lacks precision or may even be controversial. In the latter case, the system can only reflect the views of the expert whose knowledge is included. To guarantee widespread distribution of a system it is important to include a knowledge base of recognized and accepted knowledge on the one hand, and on the other hand to advise the user that in certain restricted cases the system reflects the interpretation of the expert who compiled it; thus the advice is not always consensual. The disagreement that exists between experts poses a considerable problem when evaluating information systems.

These various sources of imprecision which give rise to approximate reasonings are often mixed in the proposed formalizations. It is important to separate them because the AI methods lead to a more satisfactory solution to the problem associated with the lack of resolution implicit in unreliable techniques. They are, moreover, capable of intelligent explanation that is essential to decision-making permitting both learning and understanding of their limitations.

The possibility of approximate reasoning makes it necessary to introduce means of controlling the system, the heuristic which leads to the formulation of working hypotheses in an evocation phase where the possible hypotheses are multiple. Control is all the more important as the initial problem is vast and success depends in large part on the early generation of hypotheses by the system. Clearly, depending on the application, this approximate reasoning may be used as a simple preliminary part of the process of problem-solving based on a limited number of data, as typified by Kassirer and Gorry (1978), or even a consequential part of this process. It is followed in each case by 'categorical' reasoning which allows proposal of one or more conclusions. The system should have another fundamental property: it should be capable of initiating actions instead of just acting in response to requests from the user as many conventional systems do. This means that it must be actively controlled by the data; and in this context it should be aware of the extent of its knowledge and should thus be capable of restricting *a priori* 'the combinatorial explosion' when seeking eventual achievement of a goal. This sort of knowledge capacity is like the process of human introspection and creates heuristics such as the heuristic of evocation that has been used in SPHINX.

In the search for an appropriate formalism to represent the knowledge the dual 'declarative-procedural approach' is classic.

The two approaches need not be completely separated and the formalism adopted should be able to code knowledge in such a way that the elements handled by the system are accessible and therefore not implicitly coded, so that reasoning may be applied to them; the conditions should allow rapid access in all situations. Thus a declarative language has been used rather than a procedural language when formulating production rules to represent the knowledge. The reason for this choice lies with the modularity of the system and allows modification of data as well as having the capacity for explanation to commend it.

2
Representation and use of the knowledge

The representation of the knowledge is the main task when developing an expert system. Although, for that matter, this problem is also encountered in other areas of research such as language comprehension, robotics or intelligent data bases. In fact as the representation of the knowledge is a formalism serving as medium for the phenomena being studied, the inference capacity is powerfully influenced by the choice of representation. This choice is made initially by deciding on either procedural representation or on declarative representation. A procedural representation makes clear the relationship between the elements of knowledge whilst the declarative representation attempts to express knowledge in the form of independent 'granules' and leaves to a reasoning mechanism the grouping of the knowledge elements for making deductions (Pinson, 1981). The details of the procedures used to represent knowledge will not be gone into. It leads to the writing of programs which are difficult to modify and extend as the knowledge develops. Schematically, if one is primarily interested in declarative representation, whether pure as in production rules and the semantic network or mixed as in frames, there are two ways of approaching the problem.

Firstly, starting from predicate logic use may be made of a set of well-established mathematical results such as the principle of resolution and automated proof-solving theorems. It is now well established that predicate logic is an efficient way to represent knowledge in a declarative form.

The second approach ostensibly makes no reference to logic. The problems are tackled in various ways and we are not concerned here with the problems of resolution that the logic systems set out to solve, for example Minsky's system of frames (Minsky, 1975). Buchanan and Duda (1982) emphasize that three criteria should be met when considering knowledge representation in an expert system; namely, the extendability, the simplicity and the explicit nature of the knowledge.

1. Extendability: The data structure and the programs should be flexible enough to allow extension of the knowledge base without requiring serious revisions of the program.
2. Simplicity: Representation, like the expression of knowledge, should be simple to a non-computer expert.

   There are two ways in which conceptual simplicity can be maintained, by making the knowledge as homogeneous as possible or by writing special access functions for non-homogeneous representations.
3. Explicitness of the knowledge: This is an important element in the search for errors and the phrasing of the explanations by the system.

The greater part of the knowledge used by artificial intelligence is directly representable by implicative expressions. If it is wished to represent these as clauses of first order logic, the basic elements of which are listed in Appendix 1, the 'control' information is lost while formulating the implication. For example, clause A v. B is logically equivalent to:

$$\daleth A \rightarrow B$$
$$\daleth B \rightarrow A$$

Yet, each of these implications carries different information which no longer appears in the clausal form. The use of the rules containing the implications in a production system leads to production of inferences which stem uniquely from these rules. Each inference obtained operates one rule at a time. This limitation compared with the resolution using logic formulae generally improves efficiency of the system and makes the machine process comprehensible to the user.

2.1 PRODUCTION SYSTEMS

Production systems were proposed by Post (1943) as a general method of computation. Many expert systems are based on use of deduction rules and the expert knowledge is represented by a large number of simple rules which conduct a dialogue between the system and user in order to reach a conclusion. This computational scheme using production rules is the converse of procedural systems in practice, although, strictly speaking, they are equivalent.

2.1.1 Description of a production system

Production systems can be simplified using three basic elements, namely:

1. A collection of rules forming the knowledge base.
2. A data base (or fact base).
3. An inference engine for interpreting the rules.

The rules are assertions presented in the form of implications that may equally be thought of as conditions to be achieved for triggering a given action. They are the expression of a general knowledge in the form:

> *If* ⟨conditions⟩ *Then* ⟨actions⟩
> or *If* $A_∧ B_∧ \ldots {}_∧ G$ *Then* $H_{1∧} H_2$

Activation of the rules forms a chain of actions produced by modus ponens. The organization and the access to these rules are very important. Access can vary from a very simple scheme in which the rules are used in a predetermined order, to more complex arrangements which integrate and lead to the resolutions of conflicts. This is a dynamic method of selecting the activation of a particular rule. Broadly speaking, a rule is evaluated by reference to the content of the data base.

The data base forms the short-term memory of the program and is called either the facts base or sometimes the work space. It contains the facts, which are assertions not expressed in an implicative form. They represent knowledge calling attention to the particular case of, say, need for treatment, which might be supplied by the system or even deduced by it.

The user demonstrates a goal from the facts of data base and the knowledge rules base which is done by pattern matching (Waterman and Hayes-Roth, 1978). This automated demonstration allows the different processes to be followed making it easier for the user to understand as shown by the example Figure 2.1. This demonstrates the three phases which are typical of the use of production rules by the user who controls the order of the successive deductions; they correspond to the plan shown in Figure 2.2 (Laurière, 1982).

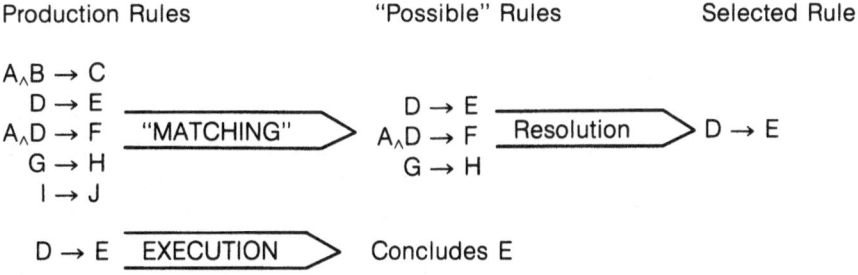

Production Rules   "Possible" Rules   Selected Rule

$A_∧B → C$
$D → E$
$A_∧D → F$ "MATCHING" ⟩ $D → E$
$G → H$ $A_∧D → F$ Resolution ⟩ $D → E$
$I → J$ $G → H$

$D → E$ EXECUTION ⟩ Concludes E

Fig. 2.1 Content of facts base.

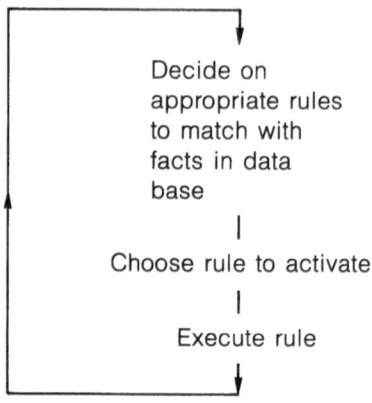

Decide on
appropriate rules
to match with
facts in data
base

Choose rule to activate

Execute rule

Fig. 2.2

The production rules technique allows expression of knowledge in a purely declarative way in a modular fashion. This is the opposite of the procedural approach which is algorithmic in nature and whose reasoning is generally neither very clear nor accessible to the user. In addition the production rules systems are sensitive to changes in state of the system. In fact, the actions may modify the data base which in turn affects the selection of the subsequent rule to be triggered.

It is of interest that the two viewpoints, cognitive psychology modelling and the production of expert systems, using respectively general problem solving techniques and systems such as MYCIN or DENDRAL, to quote just two, arrive at similar end points and use production rules. In fact Newell and Simon consider these systems as a good way of modelling cognitive processes because they are widely applicable like TURING'S machine; they allow the introduction of large numbers of new rules, and the production rules may be a possible model for long-term human memory.

Backward chaining systems

In a general way the search for the desired goal develops like the automatic proof-solving theorem. It can be represented by a deduction tree as shown in Figure 2.3. Such a deduction tree can be gone through in either direction. The principle of backward chaining is that it takes a course through the tree from the goal towards the elementary facts that sustain it. The system searches for properties which give sufficient proof to achieve the desired conclusion. It is a classical procedure for decomposing goals into sub-goals. It evaluates the premises of all the rules

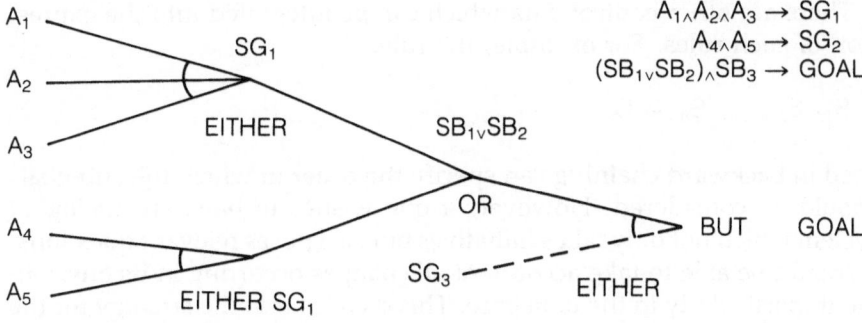

Fig. 2.3   EITHER/OR TREE; SG = sub-goal.

which return the selected goal, and to that end recursively creates the sub-aims. The moment the sub-goals are proved the process stops and the goal is attained. The rules triggered in this way are called consequent rules. The backward chaining process limits the number of premises to be evaluated and reduces the size of the tree, thus making the system more efficient since fewer conclusions are considered *a priori*.

Forward chaining systems

The premise of a rule in this case is evaluated as soon as possible for the system applies only the rules that are applicable. Properties are sought by deduction from the facts and added on as new facts. The triggering of the rules corresponds to a run through the tree in Figure 2.3. The rules triggered in this way are called antecedent rules.

2.1.2   The control structure in a production rules system

Clearly the very expression production rules knowledge implies a control element and the way the rule is applied is of prime importance. For example, rules are disposed which represent inclusion relations such as 'Hashimoto's thyroiditis is an auto-immune disease'. In this case, and all other auto-immune disease, it may be very disadvantageous to use them in forward chaining, that is to say, the reasoning ought if possible to reduce the number of alternatives. If it is known that a goitre accompanied by symptoms of hyperthyroidism is due to Hashimoto's thyroiditis we know from the outcome that it is an auto-immune disease. To follow the hierarchy in this direction does not lead to the combinational explosion. On the other hand, the counter-assumption of the preceding rule: 'if the disease is not an auto-immune disease then it is not Hashimoto's thyroiditis' may be used in backward chaining.

There are other control data which can be integrated into the expression of such rules. For example, the rule:

$$S_{1\wedge}^{\wedge} S_2^{\wedge} \ldots_{\wedge} S_n \rightarrow D$$

used in backward chaining can specify the order in which the sub-goals should be considered. However, if one wishes to have an intelligent system which not only takes initiatives but also poses relevant questions, it should be able to take account of all changes occurring in its environment, particularly in the data base. This dictates that the strategy for the choice of which rule to activate, that is the resolution of conflicts, should allow these changes to be taken into account. The system then has at its disposal an elaborate control structure. In a general way, the control structures proposed for production rule systems can be classified according to the following three types:

1. An exhaustive use of the rules leading to achievement of a goal; in which case the actual control procedure is quite elementary since it does not take into account the development of the facts base. It can be useful when the research domain is small, if the production rules are weighted and if the result obtained by each rule separately can be backed up by their joint use.
2. The activation of a rule following a criterion of choice which are many and varied. For example, the choice of rule goes to the rule most frequently used or that most recently employed; or, the choice of rule may be based on the facts in the data base with priority being given to the rule that reconciles with the fact judged to be most important.
3. The control can be affected by meta-rules in when the expression of the knowledge requires, in its mode of use, that the reasoning logic is made clear through similar rules. Thereby, the same inference engine is used to reason about the knowledge at the object-level or upon the control at the meta-level. It is not always possible to reason on the control, in fact the data are often integrated into the user code which renders them implicit and inaccessible, although this capability should be sought after because of the substantial advantages of a uniform representation at all levels (Davis, 1980a). The representation of high-level knowledge in the form of meta-rules was introduced by Davis in TEIRESIAS (Davis, 1980a). This procedure was devised to act as a genuine help in the construction of the system. The meta-rules of TEIRESIAS operate through inference rules at the object-level and finish with their being used in given situations. They represent particular strategies for using the object-level knowledge, and allow, after refinement, synthesis of a list of rules leading to a

goal. In fact meta-rules actually convey a 'knowledge of the knowledge' in a better way than any syntactic scheme.

In conclusion, a general schema of a system based on production rules is presented in Figure 2.4 based on those of Hayes-Roth *et al.* (1978) and Laurière (1982).

Knowledge Base   'Working Space'

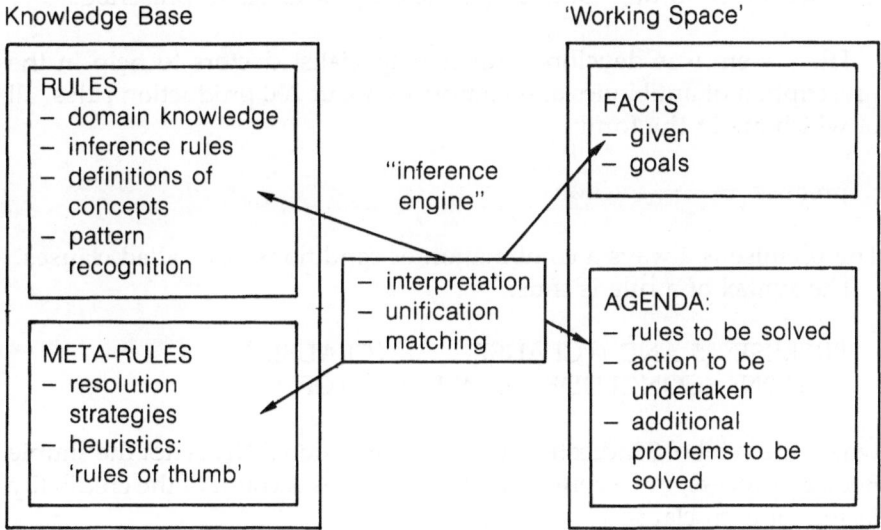

Fig. 2.4   General schema of a production rules sytem.

2.1.3   Examples of systems based on the production rules

An attempt is made to illustrate with the help of medical examples without any claim to be comprehensive how production rules methodology has been used in the provision of expert systems.

The MYCIN system (Shortliffe and Buchanan, 1975; Shortliffe, 1976)

This is a decision-making aid, originating from the group at Stanford, for identifying the micro-organisms which cause infections and also for offering therapeutic advice. The name MYCIN is derived from the suffix common to many anti-microbial drugs and reflects the aim of the program, which is to select appropriate treatment for an infection. The system does not take account of the infections caused by viruses or fungal pathogens. The process of treatment selection is broken down into four parts:

1. Does the infection require treatment?
2. If yes, identification of the organism or organisms likely to cause such infection.
3. Generation of a list of drugs which can be prescribed.
4. Selection from this list of a specific drug or drugs to prescribe.

The system was developed for non-specialist doctors to help in the prescription of antibiotics and comprises about 200 production rules, all of which are in the form:

$$\text{premise} \xrightarrow{\quad \alpha \quad} \text{action}$$

The premise is always a combination of conditions also called clauses.
   The syntax of a rule is thus:

PREMISE: (\$ AND ($\langle$CLAUSE$_1\rangle$ ... $\langle$CLAUSE$_n\rangle$)))
ACTION: (CONCLUDE $\langle$NEW FACT$\rangle$ $\langle$CF$\rangle$)

where the symbol \$ indicates that the conjunction AND is not the simple Boolean process, but a conjunction which takes account of the credibility factors of each clause.
   The 'strength' of an inference can be modified by a credibility factor (CF)α. All the MYCIN knowledge therefore presents a set of quasi-independent rules. Example of rule:

IF: — the stain is GRAM −ve
              AND
         — the morphology shows RODS
              AND
         — the patient is AT RISK
THEN: suggests (evidence 0.6) that this is a PSEUDOMONAS

α, the credibility coefficient of the rule is also called the attenuation factor of the rule and can take inclusive values between −1 and +1. Positive values express the degree of credibility consistent with the finding. As $\alpha \rightarrow 1$, the more certain the conclusion. In a similar way negative values express negative conclusions.
   The system knowledge is stored as rules without explicit reference to the way in which they are interconnected.
   The facts are represented as the members of the premises. MYCIN

utilizes quadruples to represent the data: the first three members designate the information, and the fourth is the probability value of the information:

⟨ATTRIBUTE⟩ of the ⟨OBJECT⟩ is ⟨VALUE⟩ with a certainty ⟨CF⟩

In order to find out whether a clause accords with the patient's facts base, each clause calls on a predicate which allows an exact matching to be made.

MYCIN disposes of about twenty predicates which are assessed 'TRUE' or 'FALSE' in accordance with the credibility values of the attribute.

Examples of predicates are: 'IS THE SAME AS', 'IS KNOWN', 'DEFINED'. There are eleven objects, including micro-organisms and drugs, and each is designated by a particular value of the attribute. A further example of a MYCIN rule and its LISP coding is given in Appendix 3.

MYCIN takes account of all information relevant to the patient, such as which cultures were set up and which organisms isolated; which drugs administered. Each of the entities forms a 'context' which is associated into a context tree to construct the clinical problem in each case. For example:

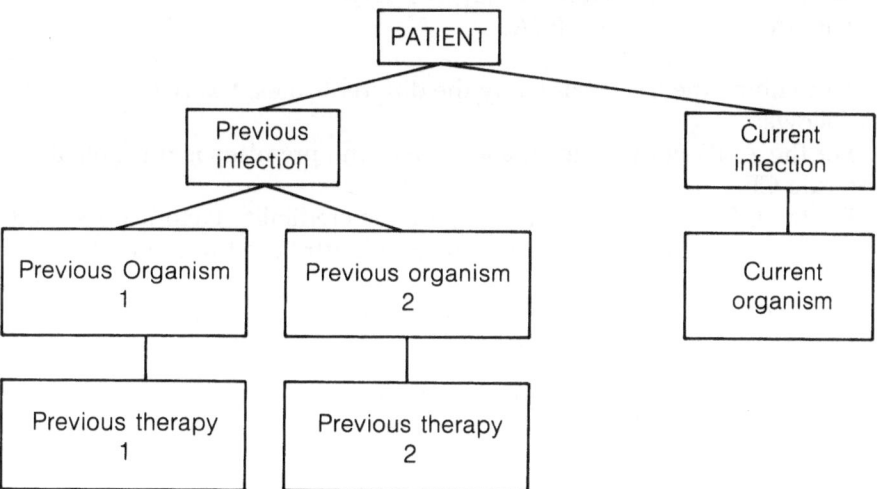

The contexts tree is actively produced during the course of the verbal consultation. To each context is attached a set of rules which will be triggered if the context is produced. This has the effect of restricting the number of rules applicable at a given instant.

MYCIN reasoning depends mainly on three components:

1. Construction of a contexts tree.
2. Construction of AND/OR trees which express the reasoning itself.
3. The meta-rules.

The contexts tree forms the data base. It is an instantiation, characteristic of the patient, of the general tree.

The diagnosis and therapy is investigated using a goal-directed control structure, that is, by a method of reverse chaining.

Using a knowledge rule the end goal is to separate its premises into sub-goals. Evaluation of the credibility factor (CF) associated with the end objective is accomplished as described in the latest version of MYCIN operating as EMYCIN (Van Melle, 1980):

For a given rule, such as $A \rightarrow B$, if A is uncertain, the attenuation factor of the rule is reduced by multiplying it by the credibility factor of A given by the user if it is positive (if not, the rule is considered inapplicable and ignored). In general, in a rule like $A \rightarrow B$, A is a logical function bringing in the operators AND and OR. The credibility, CF, of the premises is then calculated as follows:

$$CF (A_1 \text{ OR } A_2) = \max CF (A_1), CF (A_2)$$
$$CF (A_1 \text{ AND } A_2) = \min CF (A_1), CF (A_2)$$
$$CF (\neg A) = -CF (A)$$

To combine the CF obtained by the different rules, EMYCIN proceeds as follows:

For the AND nodes: the smallest CF of the premises is multiplied by the rule CF.

For the OR nodes: if CF_1 and CF_2 are the credibility factors associated with the elements of OR and CF the result attributed to node OR

$$CF = \begin{cases} CF_1 + CF_2 - CF_1 . CF_2 \text{ if CF, and } CF_2 \text{ are positive} & (1) \\ \dfrac{CF_1 + CF_2}{1 - \text{Min } CF_1, CF_2} \text{ if } CF_1 . CF_2 \ 0 & (2) \\ -(1CF_1 + 1CF_2 - CF_1 . CF_2) \text{ if } CF_1 \text{ and } CF_2 \text{ are negative} & (3) \end{cases}$$

Ishizuka *et al.* (1981) proposed a theoretical treatment of credibility factors: the main elements and the connection with the probabilities will be found in Appendix 4.

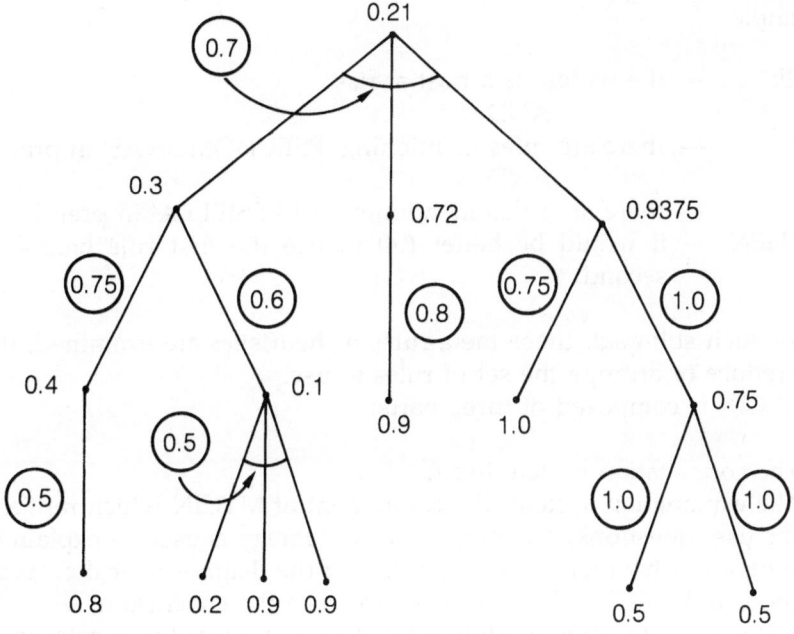

Fig. 2.5

So, where two rules have the same conclusion they are strengthened as shown in the example in Figure 2.5. The surrounding numbers designate the rules associated with CF and those underlined are the CF values allocated by the user to the various elements of the premises. It is observed that when the CF is less than 0.2 the result is classed as zero. This heuristic allows one to ignore some branches of the AND/OR tree, as well as to save time, to produce some comprehensible and less confused explanations of the system.

It should be noted that for commutative reasons, MYCIN can develop the equivalent of two AND/OR trees for a given goal, depending on which rules are present: one concerns the rules with positive CF and the other those with negative CF. On that account, equation (2) is applied once and once only to evaluate the final CF of a goal.

The system uses all the rules in turn to reach a given goal. The patient data are entered solely on request, because the system is strictly goal-directed. The user may not give data spontaneously to the system which introduces a constraint to the clinician's voluntary expression.

The third main reasoning element of MYCIN is made up of the strategy rules, or meta-rules.

Example:

> IF: — the patient is a host at risk
>   AND
>   — there are rules mentioning 'PSEUDOMONAS' in premise
>   AND
>   — there are rules mentioning 'KLEBSIELLA' in premise
> THEN: — it would be better (.4) to use the first rule before the second.

For each sub-goal, these meta-rules or heuristics are examined; they can reduce or arrange the set of rules to use.

MYCIN is composed of three parts:

1. The consultation system itself.
2. The explanation system: the component of MYCIN which replies to the user questions. The goal-directed strategy is used to explain the program behaviour in the resolution of the diagnostic or therapeutic problem by listing the rules used to reach the conclusion.
3. The rules acquisition module which takes account of new rules or the modification of existing rules.

Although the efficacy of MYCIN as a clinical tool has not been demonstrated as far as we know, it produces reliable diagnostic and therapeutic advice.

MYCIN is currently used in EMYCIN (Van Melle, 1980) which has led to other applications: PUFF (Kunz, 1978) provides interpretation of the results of functional respiratory exploration; HEADMED (Heiser and Brooks, 1978) is a psycho-pharmacological application in practical psychiatry; CLOT (Bennett, 1980) applies to problems of coagulation. EMYCIN is an expert knowledge entirely independent of the application domain. It was developed from MYCIN which comprised code sequences referred particularly to antibiotic therapy. It is equipped with a rules compiler which converts the production rules into a decision tree, eliminating redundant calculations inherent in the rules interpreter, and compiles the resulting tree in practicable code. In other words the format of the production rules is used for the acquisition of rules or is used by the explanatory module whilst the consultation module uses an effectual decision-making program. In addition, MYCIN can use antecedent rules which have the same structure as the consequent rules but differ in their use. So, each time the system has assessed a parameter it looks for the list of the antecedent rules in which this parameter appears as premise; and it applies the one whose premises are fully known. These rules never induce questions to the user. EMYCIN introduces the more extensive use of meta-rules and also provides a debugging module which is based on part of the TEIRESIAS program (Davis, 1980a); this guides the expert along the chain of reasoning and leads him to identify incorrect or missing rules.

The VM System (Fagan et al., 1979)

VM is an expert system developed from MYCIN for monitoring ventilation. It is confined to the interpretation of quantitative data collected from the intensive care unit, which are used to pilot an artificial respirator. Although strongly influenced by MYCIN, the program has been adapted to take account of the elements developing in the process of time. There are four main steps:

1. To detect the main errors of measurement.
2. To trigger signals for detection of particular events concerning either the patient or the machine itself.
3. To sum up the state of the patient.
4. To suggest therapy changes.

The system provides a model of the different stages followed by a patient, from his admission until his discharge from the intensive care service, and interpretation of the measures carried out on the patient depending on his clinical condition. In the same way, the goals proposed by the system are laid down according to the clinical context.

The knowledge is represented in the form of production rules similar to those of MYCIN. The small number of data to process allows use of an inference engine which triggers the rules in forward chaining.

Example of VM rules:

IF: the cardiac rate is acceptable
       the cardiac rate has not changed by more than 20 pulsations/min for 15 minutes
       the mean arterial pressure is acceptable
       the mean arterial pressure has not changed by more than 15 torr in 15 minutes
       the systolic pressure is acceptable
THEN: stable haemodynamics
       'Acceptable' varies in the context of the type of ventilatory aid.

The GUIDON System (Clancey, 1979), NEOMYCIN
(Clancey and Letsinger, 1981)

GUIDON was developed to evaluate the educational potential of MYCIN. MYCIN knowledge is used through teaching rules. The research strategy cannot be blind as in MYCIN. This has led to revision of existing rules to increase the knowledge by adding such concepts as: At what point should meningitis be considered? What other disease(s) could it be confused with?

The system works in the following way: a case is presented to the student in a concise and general way giving the patient's age and sex and the location of the infection; the student then asks questions about the patient with a view to making a prescription. GUIDON compares the student's questions with those put by MYCIN, assesses their relevance and examines them critically, basing its argument on the MYCIN process. Besides an expert knowledge the system has a teaching knowledge which considers the achievement of the student in four stages: beginner, advanced student, practitioner, or expert. GUIDON readjusts the skill level of the student from the results and registers them for each session in which the student plays the part of medical consultant. In addition, it uses the teaching production rules to choose a teaching goal for the session; that is, the expert knowledge which will be the aim of the lesson. This aid to the student is facilitated by the fact that the system is goal-directed, but it should be stressed that only one goal at a time is considered during the dialogue. Data which are not used by the rules to reach the goal are declared inappropriate, which in our view leads to an inflexibility in the system behaviour which may introduce constraint into a teaching experiment. However, the advantage of such systems is indubitable if only because they permit testing of the patient's signs with various research strategies. For example, to help the student, it might be suggested that he use the rule which most closely confirms a diagnosis or a therapy, or, that he use the rules which best show up its weaknesses.

The second version of the system, called NEOMYCIN (Clancey and Letsinger, 1981), uses a knowledge which has been completely rewritten and extended, the rules developed mainly in forward chaining and control ensured by a set of explicit meta-rules.

The SAM System (Gascuel, 1981)

SAM is based on the use of production rules and an approximate inference mechanism identical to MYCIN, and has been used in the treatment of hypertension and cerebrovascular accidents. The knowledge universally accepted is expressed in the form of tautologies.

Example:

Ischaemia and haemorrhage constitute cerebral vascular accidents.

Two types of reasoning are conducted in parallel by an inference engine which proceeds in forward chaining: an approximate reasoning based on the rules and a reasoning based on the tautologies. Each rule is unified once only; and the mode of use of the tautologies is rigidly defined. It is emphasized that the system does not initiate a consultation dialogue but gives advice on a pre-checked and pre-recorded medical case-history.

2.2 SEMANTIC NETWORKS

2.2.1 General presentation

Davis and King (1977) have emphasized that production rules are an attractive formalism for representing knowledge which expresses judgements, but that it is not natural to use this formalism to represent declarative knowledge, such as relations between different objects of a domain; for example, property relations which interpret a classification. Some investigators have tried to find alternative ways to present data. Early work (Quillian, 1968) was on a formalism representing the 'semantic memory'. The meaning of the words is represented with the help of a graph composed of nodes which refer to concepts linked together by various relationships; for example, bonds of homonymy and of qualification.

A semantic network is a graph in which the 'nodes' represent entities, individuals, situations and where the 'orientated arcs' are instances of 'binary relations' (the nodes play the part of terms; and the arcs the role of the predicates in logic). The network represents the set of binary assertions.

Example:

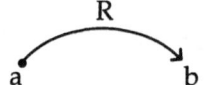

represents the assertion R (a, b)

The attraction of such a representation of the declarative knowledge derives from several points (Hendrix, 1978):

1. The semantic networks allow coding of the facts or concepts representable in any alternative formal system. They introduce a represen-

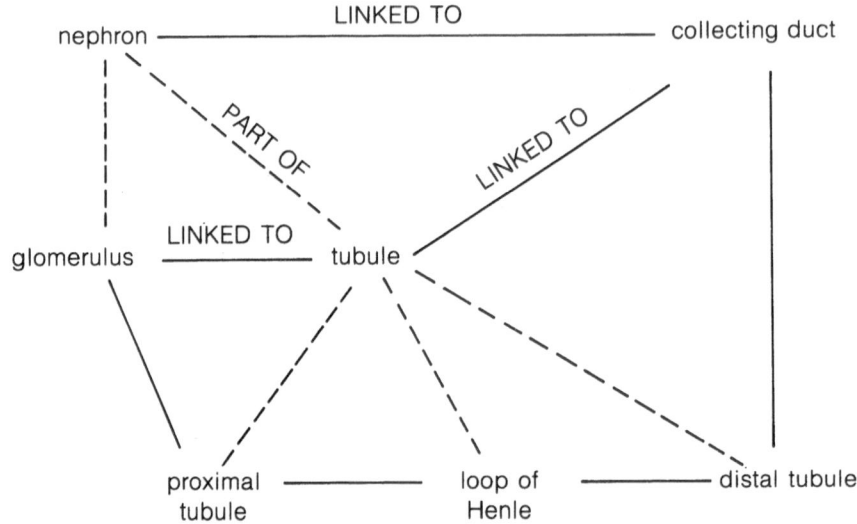

Fig. 2.6 Anatomical knowledge relating to the kidney.

tation discipline by making it obligatory to express the knowledge in binary relations from rather than in the n-ary form of relation (binary relations are attractive particularly if one wants to add information to an n-uplet).

2. They provide a very useful scheme for storing information.

Each individual is represented by a single node and all relevant assertions are directly accessible via the arcs which are connected to this node. The structures of the encoded data can serve to direct data research.

For example, anatomical knowledge can be expressed by a graph Figure 2.6. The links are not all of the same type (Patil, 1981) and it may be useful to use causal, temporal, taxonomic, associative relations, etc.

2.2.2 Examples of systems which use the semantic networks

Several systems use this method of knowledge representation although it is not always used on its own.

The best known example is PROSPECTOR (Duda *et al.*, 1977), an expert system in geology which calls on the production rules and the semantic networks. Two similar examples of medical systems are given.

The CASNET System (Weiss et al., 1978b)

This system produced at Rutgers University (New Jersey) by Weiss and Kulikowski's group has been used as a diagnostic and therapeutic aid in glaucoma. This approach to diagnostic modelling employs a semantic network of causality. The medical knowledge is represented as a network of physiological and physio-pathological states. The use of this type of knowledge gives better understanding of the mechanisms and development of the disease. However, the system does not have the capacity to use diagnostic hypotheses to direct its enquiry. It separates the process of data acquisition from that of the diagnosis. Patient symptoms are acquired by confirming (or rejecting) the states in the causal network. During this phase the system does not try to identify the diseases causing these pathological states. The diagnostic stage begins after data acquisition has been completed. It must be admitted that the authors chose a well-defined subject for this application in which physio-pathological mechanisms are well known. It is much easier to construct a causal network for glaucoma than for other diagnostic problems which makes this technique difficult to apply in other medical domains. A schema borrowed from Weiss shows the four constituent parts of CASNET (Figure 2.7) in which can be singled out:

1. Observations on the patient (signs, symptoms, examination results) which are bound by certain constraints: for example, an examination result is only available if the examination has been carried out.
2. Pathological states which portray abnormal mechanisms which may be the direct cause of the observed phenomena. They can be linked by a causal network of the form $E_i \xrightarrow{a_{ij}} E_j$ where a_{ij} expresses how a cause E_i could lead to the effect E_j.
3. Disease states defined as an upper abstraction limit.
4. Therapeutic states composed of sets of treatments linked together by constraints of interaction, of toxicity, etc.

CASNET uses 'classification tables' to reach its conclusions which are made up of rules arranged in the form:

$$B(E_i) \rightarrow D_x$$

where $B(E_i)$ is a Boolean combination of states and D_x the diagnosis.

The general diagnostic strategy is implemented by interpretation of patient observations in terms of underlying pathological states. Each state is regarded as a likely hypothesis for the patient the signs being considered under three logical headings (true, false, undecided). To evaluate the E_i states to which it is linked, each sign is weighed in a description given in rules form: The various representation levels of CASNET from Kulikowski and Weiss (1982)

$$B(S_i) \xrightarrow{Q_{ij}} E_j$$

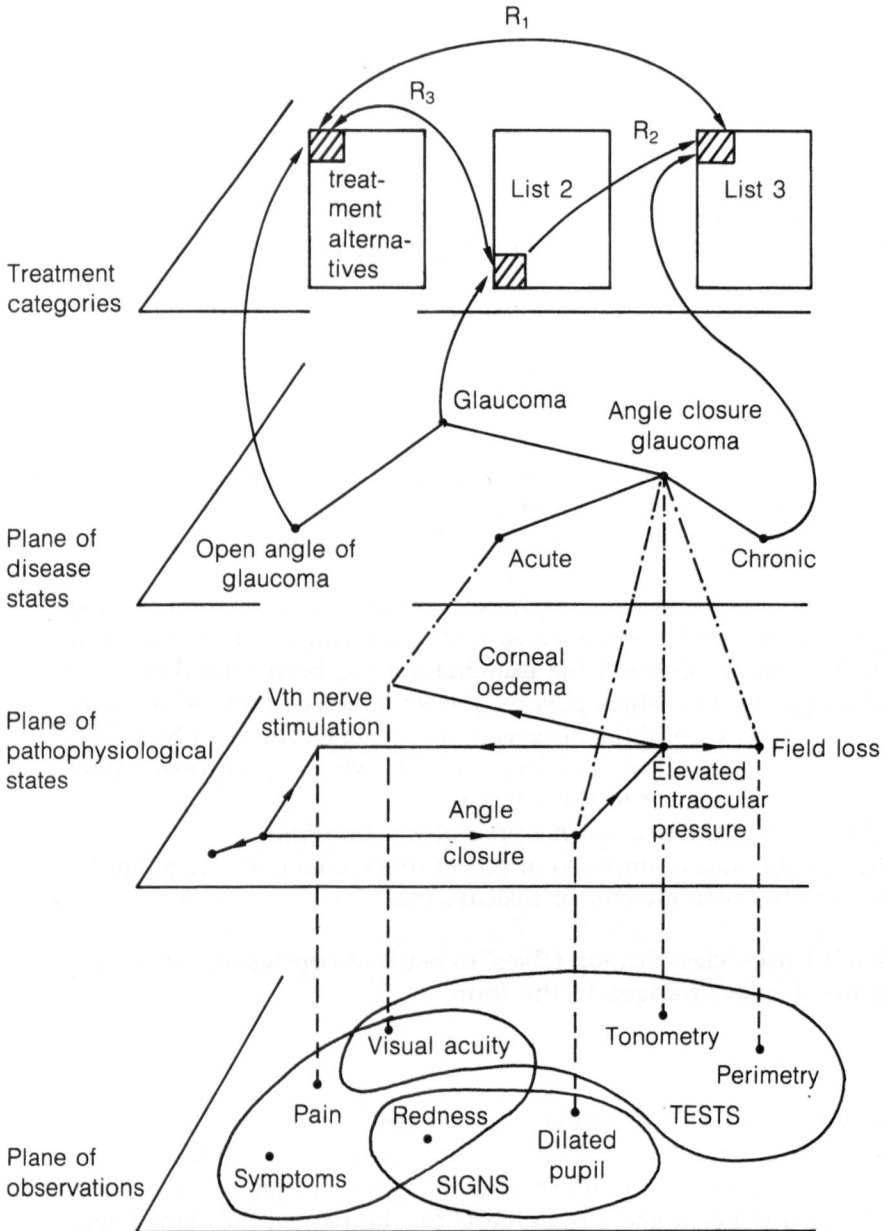

Fig. 2.7 The levels of description of disease in CASNET (from Kulikowski and Weiss, 1982).

Q_{ij} is a confidence factor associated with the causal link described. If several rules are applicable, the one with the greatest absolute value of Q_{ij} is employed to affirm or reject the state. Each patient has a set of states which may be either confirmed, rejected or undetermined. The basic states give the main causes of the disease; and starting from these states one looks for all those which can be causally linked to them by causality. Each 'base state' is connected by pointer to the relevant classification tables. The rules for disease definition are stored in order of increasing seriousness.

It is important to stress that this form of modelling does not consider diagnosis as a simple allocation to a pre-established class of patients. The patient's state is dynamically reassessed with each visit and signs of change observed.

Judging by its performance, 95% of specialists in ophthalmology favoured this system as much for its applicability as a research tool in glaucoma as for its diagnostic competence.

The CASNET system has been generalized and extended in a version called EXPERT (Kulikowski and Weiss, 1982). It has been applied to micro-processors, one of which is marketed as CLINISCAN; this apparatus elicits blood protein electrophoresis results and interprets them (Kulikowski *et al.*, 1981).

The ABEL System (Patil, 1981)

ABEL was developed to study the benefit and use of representations depicting hierarchical causal links in diagnostic and therapeutic reasoning in the domain of water and electrolyte disorders. The authors have developed a schema of hierarchical representation to describe the medical knowledge and procedures which can be substantiated for a particular disease. The lowest level consists of a physio-pathological knowledge which is successively assembled into higher level concepts and relations passing gradually from physiological description to a more comprehensive 'syndrome' knowledge, allowing a more effective examination of the diagnostic goal. The physiological knowledge makes it possible to deal with complex clinical situations. Moreover, causal physiological reasoning is by its nature unquestionable in contrast with reasoning which depends on approximate, even probable syndromes. The hierarchic description permits use of the two reasonings at a time. The authors distinguish five different representation levels, each of which can be seen as a semantic network showing the relations between different states. Each node of the network is associated with a set of attributes of time, severity, etc. A node is called composite if it can be appointed in causal terms to a more detailed level, otherwise it is a primitive node.

Example:
Elaboration of a causal link between DIARRHOEA and DEHYDRATION

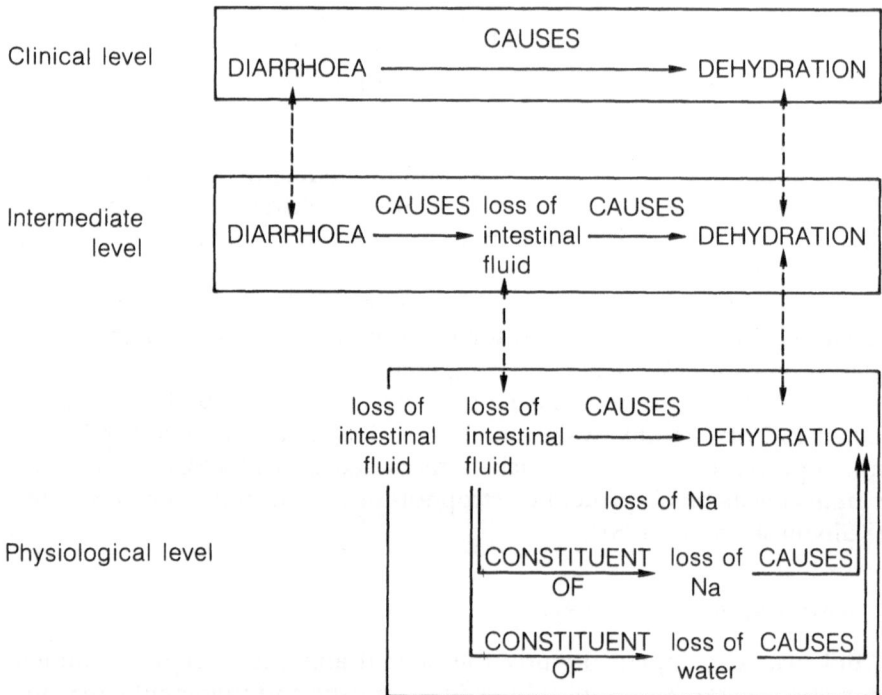

For each possible explanation of a patient's state, ABEL constructs a specific model as procedural aid. Thus, from initial data the system assembles some possible models which explain the diagnosis. This initial construction is made from the analysis of known electrolyte results. It leads to formulation of all the acid-base disorders which are in agreement with the given electrolyte values. The system then follows three procedures: aggregation, elaboration and projection.

Aggregation is a summary of patient particulars at a higher level than the one given, and effected if the system realizes that a causal network node, for a number of reasons, is put at a higher level by a single node.

Elaboration is the twofold process of the aggregation. It depicts a causal network at a given level of detail after passing from a less detailed level; this involves disintegration of a network description.

The process of projection is used to make the hypotheses and to explain the conclusions suggested by the states of the various models. It is similar to the elaboration but differs from it by the fact that the proposed causal relationship is hypothetical and therefore not present in the patient model. This procedure is a check on whether the hypothesis representation includes inconsistency in any level of aggregation and its application allows examination of the diagnostic possibilities.

A significant concept has been introduced to the level of primitive nodes in the network. A primitive node can have components which are other primitive nodes. This arrangement is achieved by two operators:

1. Summation of the components.
2. Decomposition of components.

These operators lead to assignment, for example, of only part of the hypokalaemia to diarrhoea and to calculate what percentage of the hypokalaemia is not caused by the diarrhoea. It therefore allows analyses of complex phenomena making them easier to identify and understand.

This model lends itself to close examination of the subtlety and abundance of the knowledge and the hypotheses employed by the experts. In fact, the causal relationships play a central role in identifying diagnostic classes since presence or absence of a causal connection between two states can change their diagnostic and prognostic inter-pretation. Beyond the hierarchical representation at several levels, the main aim is to provide the system with the capacity to hypothesize the presence or absence of a causality link between two phenomena. There is then the need to be able to 'manipulate' these links like real objects to work on and not simply pointers between the nodes of a network.

2.3 FRAMES (MINSKY, 1975)

2.3.1 General presentation

Minsky introduced the idea that we have in our memory stereotyped information structures from which a choice is made each time a new situation occurs, one of these stereotypes coincides with any given situation. He introduced the term 'Frames' to combine a number of con-cepts about knowledge representation. Frames were considered as an alternative to the semantic networks and to the computation of the predicates allowing a mixed knowledge of declarative and procedural representations, which provides considerable flexibility.

A frame is a data structure; an 'expression' which represents a situation type or stereotype. Frames may be considered as a generalization of the networks where the elements or objects are more complex. A frame contains slots which can be frames themselves or simple detectors. For example, one might have a frame representing a case with slots called

History, Physical Examination, Family History, Laboratory Tests. A particular case is therefore an instantiation of the frame case obtained by filling up the slots corresponding to the disease in question. Each instantiated frame refers to one individual and each slot refers to a relation. Seen in this way frames are essentially sets of properties. The main part of a frame represents entities composed of *attributes* associated with markers which show, on one hand, the way each attribute is produced and, on the other, the tasks to be performed when an attribute has been produced. These tasks might be, for example, the production of pre-recorded attributes. Thus, suppose that the frame 'identity' comprises the characteristics of 'age' and 'sex'. If the patient is male and aged forty it is natural to assume that his weight and height (two factors belonging to other frames) lie between certain limits; it may be assumed that the weight of this man is very likely to be between 50 and 110 kg and his height between 1.55 m and 1.90 m. 'Weight' and 'height' are therefore affected by the attributes of age and sex in the frame 'identity'.

The use of frames to represent knowledge requires two processes: the first, which is goal-directed, assigns a value to an attribute; and the second and predominant one is data-directed to accomplish the necessary task. Attachment to the attributes of procedures triggered following their evaluation is an important property of the frames; there are two recognizable classes of procedure:

1. Domestic procedures or 'servants', triggered only on demand.
2. Demons, which are automatically activated as soon as a fact arrives to find a place in an instantiation of the frame.

Frames can describe and represent all aspects of a given situation and are usually linked together to form a frame, tree, or occasionally a network.

Certain slots can be given values in the absence of information or a slot may even be assigned a value inherited from a different frame.

Several inference rules may be used in a knowledge representation by the frames:

1. The first inference rule used is the instantiation. Given a frame which represents a concept, the concept may be instantiated by filling the slots.
2. A further inference rule was suggested by MINSKY. It is explicitly implemented in certain frames applications: the 'criteriality inference' (Hayes, 1981). If all the slots of a frame are filled it may be inferred from this rule that the concept is instantiated by the frame; for example, if an entity is equipped with interrogation, and clinical

examination results, it may be a patient (possession of these attributes is sufficient to qualify the patient). One example of use of this rule is through perceptive reasoning: if it is intended to identify an X-ray of the thorax and all the pertinent slots are filled, then it can be stated that a thorax X-ray is identified.

Representation in first order logic of a frame establishes the concept C with the relations R_1, R_2 ... R_n as follows:

$$\forall x C(x) = \exists y_1 \ldots \exists y_n R_1(x, y_1) \wedge \ldots \wedge R_n(x, y_n)$$

or put into clausal form:

$$\forall x C(x) \rightarrow R_1(x, f_1(x))$$

$$_\wedge \forall x C(x) \rightarrow R_2(x, f_2(x))$$

$$_\wedge \forall X C(X) \rightarrow R_n(x, f_n(x))$$

$$_\wedge \forall x, \forall y_1 \ldots \forall y_n R_1(x, y_1) _\wedge R_2(x, y_2) \ldots _\wedge R_n(x, y_n) \rightarrow C(x)$$

where the final clause explicitly expresses the criteriality inference.

2.3.2   Examples of systems using the frames

The INTERNIST system (Pople et al., 1975)

INTERNIST is a diagnostic aid program which deals with about 80% of hospital medicine through application of the most comprehensive and the greatest number of rules: it comprises three to four thousand manifestations of five hundred different diseases!

The INTERNIST data base associates with each possible diagnosis D_i a set of manifestations m_j. A manifestation is a sign, a symptom, a laboratory result or other associated diagnosis. The system is built up from various hierarchical classifications by successively weighing up different classes of pathology such as diseases of the liver, heart, etc. The subcategories are selected for the similarity of their pathogenic mechanisms.

The use of hierarchies is an important means of controlling the proliferation of the working hypotheses during a consultation.

The authors single out three important relations which influence the use of the medical knowledge base:

1. The EVOKE relation (M, D) which makes apparent the association between manifestation M and disease D.

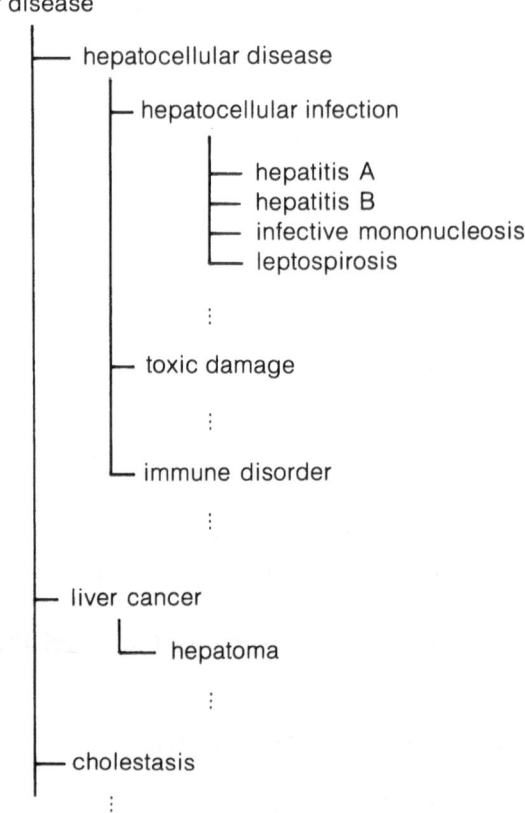

liver disease
— hepatocellular disease
— hepatocellular infection
— hepatitis A
— hepatitis B
— infective mononucleosis
— leptospirosis
⋮
— toxic damage
⋮
— immune disorder
⋮
— liver cancer
— hepatoma
⋮
— cholestasis
⋮

2. The FORM-OF connection (D_1, D_{1-1}) which affirms that the disease D_{1-1} is a form of disease D_1; for example, D_{1-1} may be hepatitis A and D_1 a liver disease.
3. The MANIFEST connection (D, M) which is the inverse relation of EVOQUE between the disease and its manifestation.

Using these predicates:

$$\forall d\,(\text{FORM-OF}\;(D_1, d) \rightarrow \text{MANIFEST}\,(d, M_1))$$

that is all diseases of a certain category D_1 may show the same manifestation M_1.

By reason of the large number of data, explicit networks are used to code the disease hierarchies (see Figure 2.8).

For each M_j and the D_i, the system provides two elements for calculating the probability of the hypothesis D_i:

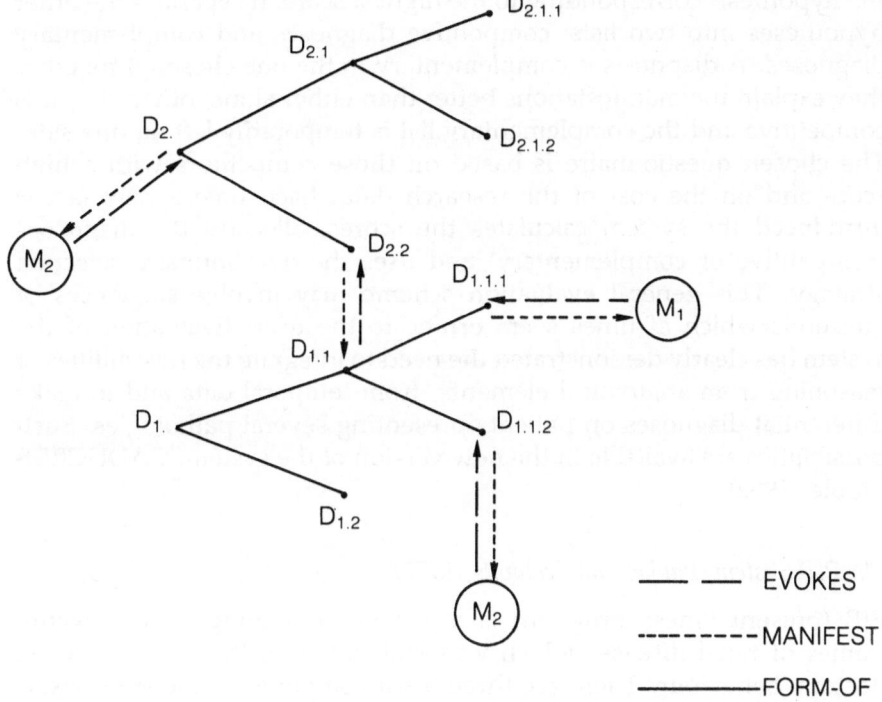

Fig. 2.8 Example of links between the knowledge elements in INTERNIST.

1. The evocation capability L_{D_i/M_j}; with coefficient between 0 and 5, which shows how the diagnosis D_i may cause the manifestation M_j. If the evocation value is equal to 0 then the manifestation is atypical of the disease D_i; whereas, the value 5 means that M_j is pathognomonic with D_i.
2. The coefficient F_{M_j/D_i} is an estimation of the frequency of the diagnoses D_i where the sign M_j is present.

A diagnosis will be active if at least one of these signs has been observed. For each active hypothesis the system works out a score from the sum of the evocation capacities of all the signs adding bonus points for diagnoses linked by cause and effect and substracting coefficients F_{M_j/D_i} for M_j's not found in the patient.

The concept according to which all diseases of a certain type share a common manifestation is recorded on the network by the MANIFEST and EVOKE links which relate to the non-terminal nodes.

The hypotheses prescribed on the basis of these scores allows continuation of the analysis. The INTERNIST system focuses research on the hypothesis corresponding to the highest score. It separates the other hypotheses into two lists: competitive diagnoses and complementary diagnoses. A diagnosis is complementary to the one chosen if together they explain the manifestations better than either alone; otherwise, it is competitive and the complementary list is temporarily left on one side. The chosen questionnaire is based on those competitors with a high score and on the cost of the research data. Each time a new fact is introduced the system calculates the scores, allocates the diagnoses (competitive or complementary) and uses the questionnaire selection strategy. This general evaluation scheme may involve sequences of questions which at times seem erratic to the user. Evaluation of the system has clearly demonstrated the need to integrate the possibilities of reasoning from anatomical elements, from temporal data and to make differential diagnoses on patients presenting several pathologies. Such possibilities are available in the new version of the system, CADUCEUS (Pople, 1982).

The PIP System (Pauker and Szolovits, 1977)

PIP (present illness program) is a system containing about seventy frames of renal diseases which was built up from the analysis of the doctors' behaviour. There are three main components; the supervisor, the short-term memory and the long-term memory. The data supplied to the system are stored in the short-term memory which also contains a certain number of 'demons' compiled taking account of the knowledge stored in the long-term memory. The demons are associated with special signs or triggers which act as a key for access to the demons; these are designated 'key signs'. If the patient data are constituent with a key sign, the corresponding diagnostic hypothesis is immediately activated, the demons are triggered, and the result is an up-date or modification of the short-term memory. These up-datings can themselves activate procedures, etc.; in particular, the demons permit activation of the diagnostic hypotheses structured in the long-term memory in the frames network form, which are so many sets of data in a small sub-set of the medical knowledge. Each of these frames may represent either a disease such as acute glomerulo-nephritis, or a clinical condition like nephrotic syndrome, or even a physio-pathological state such as sodium retention. The frames are represented by the following elements:

1. The set of signs which are typical of the disease, clinical conditions or physiopathological state.
2. The set of rules for establishing or discarding the entity in question.
3. A function allowing calculation of a probability score for the considered frame.

4. The links with other frames which are often merged with the frame described; they allow the differential diagnosis to be made.
5. The causal links to other entities which may be the cause of the entity represented by the frame.
6. The links with other entities which may complicate the pathological condition described.

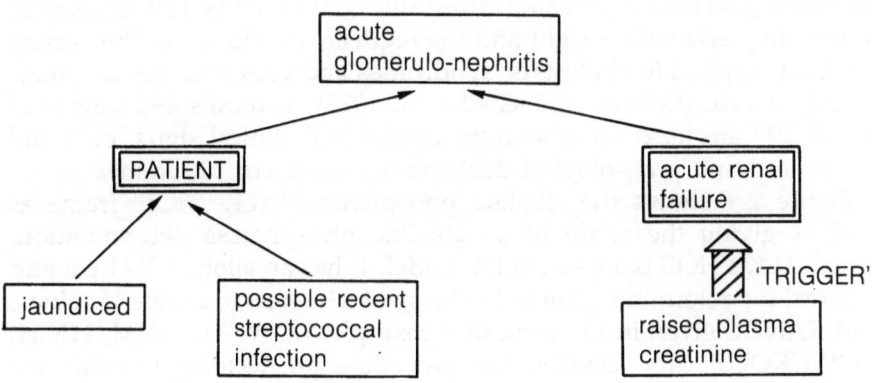

Appearance of a key sign leads to the loading into the short-term memory of the frame in which it arises. Active hypotheses are the possible explanations of the patient's state which serve as a reasoning base for the program of interrogation and research. Inactive hypotheses are those which do not arise in the reasoning either because no sign has suggested them, or because they have been considered and rejected. Entities which are related to the activated frame (by links of cause and effect for example) become semi-active hypotheses; they represent hypotheses which are not actively considered but may be the doctor's mental reservation. If the patient presents some sign which occurs in a semi-active hypothesis it becomes active, although only a key sign can activate an inactive hypothesis; so, all signs which are considered in the definition of the entity are regarded as key signs. Each hypothesis is associated with a set of complementary hypotheses whose interactions are of a causal or associative nature; or, of 'complication' type in which one pathological state is known to be a complication of another. When a hypothesis is activated all the complementary hypotheses are put into the semi-active state. PIP bases its strategy of research of the signs on the probability of the hypotheses. This probability is estimated by combination of two elements: one function measuring the suitability of the signs observed and the signs expected in the diagnostic hypothesis; and a second function connecting the signs framing the hypothesis to the total number of signs known to the system. These two compounds of the probability estimation are called 'matching score' and 'binding score'. The machine puts relevant questions to the frame with the highest score until all have been either confirmed or rejected.

The PATREC/MDX System (Mittal and Chandrasekaran, 1980)

The authors have attempted to produce an intelligent aid to management of a data base which allows versatile control of the data to respond to user requests with insight and the requisite conclusions. The system has been applied to cholestatic syndromes and uses a frames language based on FRL (Roberts and Goldstein, 1977). It recalls 490 frames of which 200 are used for laboratory results and clinical signs, etc.; and anatomical and physiological descriptions represent 150 frames.

Figure 2.9 shows the alkaline phosphatase 'ALK-PHOS' frame as well as giving the result of an alkaline phosphatase determination. Thus, ALK-PHOS is a LABDATA model. It has an allotted VALUE and NORM, for determining normal values, which refers to a scale of values, and RANGE given in the form of a sextuple: LOW, MEDIUM, HIGH, AGE GROUP, SEX, UNITS. The procedure for deciding whether the VALUE is normal or not, uses RANGE.

Part (b) of Figure 2.9 provides the information: 'The alkaline phosphatases were 14.6 Bodansky units and remained stable'.

```
       (ALK–PHOS
          (TYPE ($VALUE (LABDATA)))
          (VALUE ($VALUE...))
          (NORM ($RANGE (((21.0 52.5 85.0 (8U) ? IU) ...)))
   (a)            ($VALUE (...))
                  (FROM (VALUE)))
          (TREND ($VALUE ...)
                  (FROM (VALUE)))

       (ALK-PHOS-1
          (VALUE ($VALUE ((BU 14.6))))
   (b)    (TREND ($VALUE  (STABLE)))
          (TYPE ($VALUE (ALK-PHOS)))
          (PATIENT EPISODE ($VALUE ("ON ADMISSION")))
```

Fig. 2.9 The alkaline phosphatase "ALK–PHOS" frame and the result of an alkaline phosphatase determination.

The CENTAUR System (Aikins, 1980)

The knowledge is represented by a combination of frames and production rules. The system gives diagnostic advice on functional respiratory examination with explanation of its reasoning. The frames clarify the contexts; that is, those facts and preconditions which describe the situation and direct the use of production rules to a more discerning knowledge. The rules are therefore grouped as a function of their use in the consultation and are attached to the frames 'slots' (following Minsky's terminology).

CENTAUR uses, to explain its reasonings, frames defining broad contexts within which more detailed explanation rules are included.

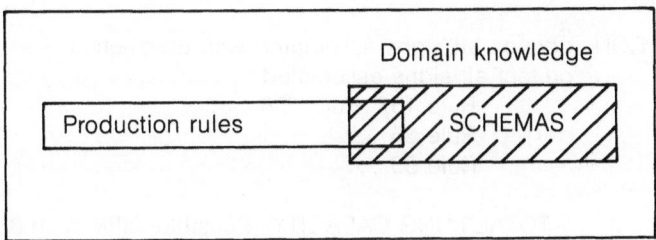

The system is based on the knowledge given in the form of production rules from PUFF (Kunz *et al.*, 1978). There are 142 of these rules using 59 clinical parameters such as age, total pulmonary capacity, etc.

General schema of a CENTAUR frame:

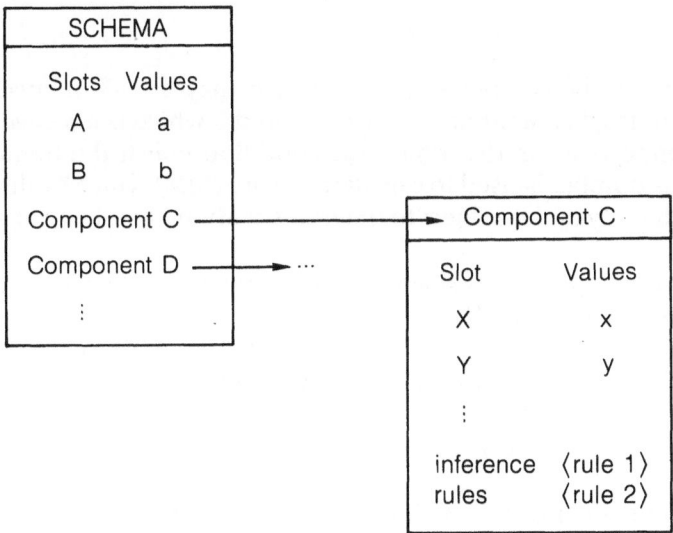

A component of CENTAUR is a slot which itself has a frame structure; an example is given in Figure 2.10.

The system puts questions to the user when there is no inference rule

OBSTRUCTIVE SYNDROME SCHEMA

* POINTS AGAINST THE: (moderate degree of
  OTHER SCHEMAS   (asthma type of
                       (emphysema . . .)

* HYPOTHESIS : AIR-WAY OBSTRUCTION

* TO CONFIRM: deduce the degree of obstruction
              deduce the type of obstruction

* ACTION: deduce all signs associated with obstruction
          protect all signs associated
                    Rule 157, Rule 158, . . .
                    Rule 36 . . .
                    Rule 53 . . .

* TOTAL LUNG CAPACITY: Possible value > 100
                       Importance of the
                       measurement: 4
* REVERSIBILITY: Inference Rule: Rule 19
                       Importance of the: 0
                       measure

Fig. 2.10   A CENTAUR frame.

for evaluating the component, or, again, if they are all in check. Each component is given a number between 1 and 5 which is a measure of its relative importance in describing the condition which the frame represents. This number is used to calculate a score (MM) which evaluates the frame suitability of the subject to the frame with the following algorithm.

For each component evaluated, if its value is reasonable —
$MM = F((100.IM)MM)$
where IM is the significance of each component measurement and F is the MYCIN-type certainty factor.
or:
$MM = F((-100.IM)MM)$

This score is compared with a threshold which decides whether the frame is confirmed or rejected. The slots 'IF CONFIRM' and 'IF REJECT' provide ways of continuing the consultation.

Besides the 'inference' rules of production used in the 'components' CENTAUR provides four types of supplementary production rules:

1. Synthesis rules which allow gross interpretation of the state of the subject.
2. Refinement rules which are used when the system has confirmed a certain number of frames; they lead on to the final diagnosis.
3. Frames activation rules which are triggered in forward chaining and lead to formulation of the hypotheses for testing.
4. 'Residual facts' rules which are applied at an advanced stage in the consultation, after confirmation or rejection of the frames, so as to be sure that the diagnosis is complete. The CENTAUR control structure is relatively straightforward: the user carries out the tasks in the order in which they appear on his agenda and stops when it is empty. The task list is modified by the activated slots; tasks remaining to be done may themselves make others necessary.

2.4 OTHER SYSTEMS

2.4.1 The XPLAIN System (Swartout, 1983)

This system is based on an automated programmer 'WRITER' which constructs a trace of the process of working out therapeutic advice in the prescription of digitalis. The trace serves as a basic document which the system provides to the user, and for which WRITER uses several types of knowledge in the domain:

1. The model of the domain which is a set of relations of cause and effect significant in digitalin therapy. It presents similarities to the CASNET networks with certain differences, for example, the causal links are not weighted. Part of the model is shown in Fig. 2.11.

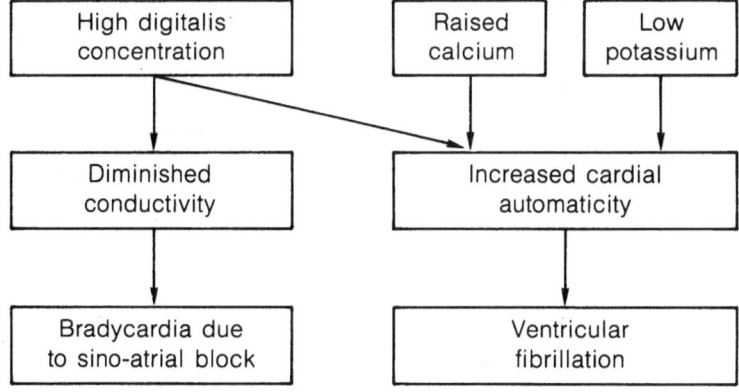

Fig. 2.11 Part of the XPLAIN Model (Swartout, 1983).

2. The principles of the domain whose knowledge express behaviour which leads to a suitable prescription. For example, for the measure intended to 'anticipate toxicity of the drug', the behaviour type is expressed as follows:

IF: clinical signs of toxicity are present
THEN: to reduce the dose
OTHERWISE: to maintain the dose

3. The refinement structure is a tree of goals decomposed into more specific sub-goals, which is produced by the WRITER program.

It provides a way of tracking through the system, and is the basis of a structure for yielding explanation. The general outline of the system is given below.

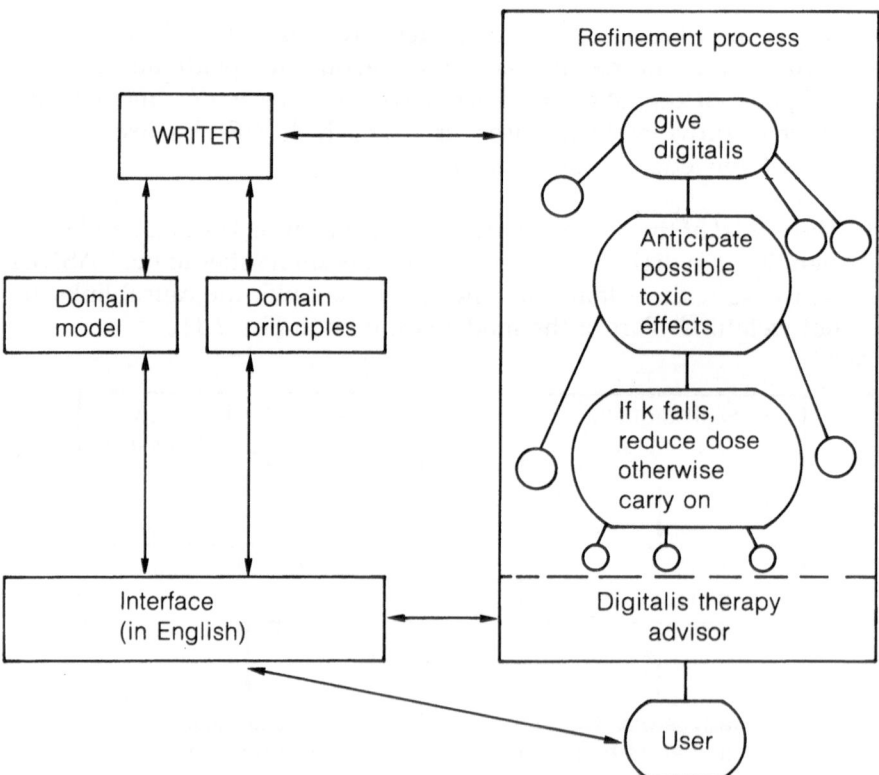

Fig. 2.12

2.4.2   ATTENDING (Miller, 1983)

In ATTENDING the system rather than making definite suggestions criticizes the management plan of the anaesthetist using ATN (Augmented Transition Networks), a natural language representation. This was the first medical system to use a critiquing approach to problems. The ATTENDING approach is 'this is what should be considered in the management of your patient'. Whereas earlier systems stated what should be done. The author emphasizes the advantage of this approach in that it enables the anaesthetist to plan patient management more effectively and in a clinically acceptable way, as the computer gives advice on improving the management plan.

2.5   DISCUSSION

The reasoning processes of the systems mentioned will now be described briefly as will the methods of knowledge representation. It is important to remember, however, that the various systems were developed for different reasons. For instance, INTERNIST was developed as a diagnostic tool; PIP attempts to emulate the behaviour of an expert in renal medicine, by simulating clinical cognition as a way to helping the non-expert to make decisions. Thus, the objectives, the underlying concepts and strategies tend to be different. Neither PIP nor INTERNIST can explain why a particular frame is activated, but CENTAUR has this ability with control by way of the 'if-confirmed' and 'if-denied' slots which specify what action is to be taken.

In PIP and INTERNIST the explicit control representation allows both systems to explain their actions and facilitates modifications to the knowledge base.

The difficulties associated with defining and understanding the complexity of a medical specialty led researchers to devise a knowledge representation that allows 'approximate reasoning'. There are several such models. For instance in MYCIN, weighted production rules are used to reach conclusions, using both 'approximate' and certain knowledge, the latter in the form of a context tree and associated rules.

INTERNIST, through the evokes-link, has the ability to determine the extent to which a finding is associated with a disease and grade the likelihood of a particular disease from a tree-like diagnostic hierarchy. It is to be noted that individual findings are able to prompt hypotheses while in CENTAUR the rules activating frames allow combinations of clinical signs to trigger a hypothesis. The tree structure is an important part of the system in controlling the possible proliferation of working hypotheses. Moreover, the progression from the general to the particular is in accord with the clinical method of the physician. Further-more, it allows the system to reach a justifiable conclusion even when information is incomplete.

Such a system, as also in PIP, follows a strategy that attempts to account for all the information presented to the system. Thus in both, incorrect information may give rise to incorrect hypotheses that are progressively more unlikely as all possible hypotheses are evoked. To overcome this, specific rules bring about termination of the consultation before this situation arises. CENTAUR contains information about likely sources of error which allows the system to recognize inconsistent or incorrect facts.

Neither PIP nor INTERNIST is a production rule system, that is clinical signs and symptons entered into the system are not acted upon by rule-based inference as in CENTAUR or MYCIN. But the problem still arises as to whether real-life situations can be reduced to a stereotypic form capable of description in such formations.

Knowledge representation in a declarative form can facilitate this, as well as allowing use of natural language for user dialogue and explana-tion. The reasoning of a system like MYCIN does not always correspond to the reasoning of the physician in that all possible solutions are explored for whenever an attribute is traced, all possible values are traced, not just that required to satisfy a particular goal. Two further points concerning a system such as MYCIN deserve mention:

1. The extent of an 'either/or' tree structure is limited compared with an individual's reasoning ability and necessitates the application domain to be broken down into problems and sub-problems.
2. Backward chaining has the advantage of allowing questioning to develop in a coherent fashion, but this coherence is a function of the tree structure rather than of the clinical domain. Indeed, a rule may depend on many differing medical facts and there may be great difficulties in maintaining a sensible 'conversational logic' in the system. Production rules may be thought of as a simple and efficient way of representing judgemental knowledge, but in fact are not suitable for describing the knowledge association with taxonomic relationships and concepts. Moreover, the diffuse structure is re-latively inefficient, the interactions between rules are not always easy to anticipate or control.
3. The composition rule of the credibility factors should be clearly understood by the expert who provides the knowledge. In fact, from the following two rules:

$$R = A \rightarrow D\ (CF_1)$$
$$R_2 = B \rightarrow D\ (CF_2)$$

MYCIN affirms D with a CF above CF_1 and CF_2 calculated from the formula $CF = CF_1 + CF_2 - CF_1 . CF_2$, if CF_1 and CF_2 are positive. It would seem that if the expert produces his knowledge on D through a single rule such as R_3, the CF' spontaneously provided by the expert will in many cases be different from the CF calculated from the other knowledge term which brings in R_1 and R_2.

$$R_3 = A_\wedge B \rightarrow D \; (CF')$$

Shortliffe (1976) has tried to show that there is quite a good correlation between the calculated CF and the CF'. However, he observes that the difference between the two increases after the combination formula has been used several times; clearly the greater the number of reasoning steps involved the more inaccurate and imprecise the result.

Although attractive in some cases the causal model is seldom used by doctors for diagnostic research (Elstein *et al.*, 1979), besides, it is difficult outside certain domains to produce or elaborate a causal network. CASNET owes its success to the fact that it has been applied in a restricted diagnostic domain where the physio-pathology is very well understood. From the more general viewpoint the single representation of links presented in the CASNET system is inadequate; in fact, it infers that all interactions between the states are of a causal nature while it is quite evident that two states may be linked in a causal way to a third, without there being any known causal link between them. CASNET, like ABEL, proposes an incomplete but interesting model of a morbid process which includes two types of knowledge: theoretical knowledge of physio-pathological mechanisms and practical knowledge of the phenomena and association of signs detected empirically. Kulikowski and Weiss (1982) describe the two model types included in CASNET:

1. A *descriptive* model which provides a description of diseases in a rather similar way to the medical textbook. Epidemiological or statistical results summarize the collected material and constitute an experimental model. Unfortunately, due to the present limits of the knowledge and the variability of definitions in medicine there are few links between the signs and intermediary states in physio-pathology.
2. A *normative* model enables characterization of the decision-making technique through decision rules by which a pathological state can be inferred, or preference for a treatment, with a degree of certainty from observed signs.

Evaluation of the degree of confidence accorded to a state is made by the operator MAX. This is calculated at each step taking the greater of two values, namely, the degree of confidence before the state and the degree of confidence which can be assigned to it when the final sign is obtained. Use of this operator, mainly employed in systems dependent on the theory of fuzzy groups, offers a particular advantage when the signs considered in the decision are not independent.

Goldberger (1982) points out that there can be no risk if a system such as CASNET were applied to such conditions as glaucoma, the thyroid diseases (Kulikowski and Ostroff, 1980) or to rheumatology (Lindberg *et al.*, 1980). In effect, these diseases are progressive and change in such a way that with passing time symptoms become evident (indicating the development or the severity of the condition) while the original signs persist. This development allows progress along the semantic networks. This model would be difficult to employ for diseases whose evolution followed a different path (a course through several phases presenting various symptomatologies).

One of the interesting facets of expert systems is their capacity for reasoning with certainty factors. This is important from a practical viewpoint as it is sometimes difficult to tell whether data are 'correct' or 'complete'. Sources of uncertainty such as missing or incorrect data, missing rules or inappropriate models, in some cases evoke reasoning mechanisms which exploit the redundancy. If some signs are redundant for reaching a conclusion it will be strengthened by them.

In conclusion, it is felt necessary to emphasize certain points:

1. The formalism used should be able to code the knowledge in such a way that the useful facts may be rapidly accessible in the appropriate situations. Explicit relations between the various facts need to be established using a uniform knowledge representation. In particular, it seems intuitive that when the conditions of a rule are true this provides information for verifying other rules which have a good chance of being true as well. This capacity does not always exist in the 'classical' production systems which operate blind, from this point of view.

2. Certain relations are occasionally allowed for in the programming because they exceed the representation capacity. As a result, the knowledge base is very soon difficult to control and its development by a non-computer operator impossible. This leads to the choice of a declarative rather than a procedural language for the modularity, the explanation possibilities and the developing characters which it procures. In addition, the introduction of procedures such as demons is burdensome since the system must be certain at all times that no demon has been introduced or triggered.

3. The representation of many concepts includes descriptions in default of information. Some assertions would be considered true unless known elements of the system led to thinking otherwise.

4. The control structure must be conceptually straightforward, capable of reasoning upon difficult problems but not too complex itself or the expert could not predict the effects of adding new rules to the knowledge. Operations on MYCIN in particular substantiate this.
5. The selected representation should allow for meta-descriptions; and the system must be capable of encoding the way in which the knowledge should be organized, used and interpreted.
6. Strategies should be sensitive to the context of the problem and expressed by meta-rules.
7. The same inference engine should be used for reasoning at both the object level and the meta-level (through the control).
8. The efficiency of an expert system is shown by its ability to use several expressions of a knowledge.

PART TWO
Study of an Expert System

3

The SPHINX system

The main aim of the SPHINX project was to provide clinicians with an information system aid to diagnostic, therapeutic or preventive decision-making, with four basic objectives:

1. The knowledge should lead the system to give advice comparable to that of an expert.
2. Dialogue with the machine should be conducted in a language as clear and as close as possible to natural language to avoid the necessity for the user to learn a particular language or code.
3. The system should potentially be able to explain its decisions by providing the elements on which it bases its reasoning.
4. In order to improve its advice, to adapt to change in medical data, and to increase its applications, the system should be equipped with a data acquisition module easy for a layman to use.

Although it is not necessary to mimic a human expert approach to produce a good program, it is confirmed, especially in medicine, that medical practice and behaviour can only be understood through interrogation of the best practitioners to discover how they tackle any particular problem. So programs are judged by reference to medical opinion and it is natural that this should lead to the development of methods which mimic medical attitudes. This leads to the development of (medical) educational systems which provide the experts with a better understanding of their subject which, in turn, improves their teaching method. In this perspective it seemed advantageous to produce a system capable of simulating a medical consultation by working out an exact copy of the behaviour of a doctor facing his patient. Just as a doctor listens to his patient to find reasons for the consultation, so the system should be capable of accepting data supplied spontaneously by the user to enable it to ask for more information, because earlier data reminds it of a diagnosis or a number of possible diagnoses. With this approach it is important to direct the research and the use of relevant data. For example, at what moment does he choose what question to ask or what sign to follow up? This stresses the point that the system should be able to initiate action when necessary rather than being directed by the user as in conventional systems. The system must be 'aware' of its data and possess an 'auto knowledge' which is not unlike human introspection. To set up such a system poses several questions:

1. How may different types of knowledge such as uncertain information or reliable data be represented?
2. How may the system be initiated through data control?
3. How may the system-user interaction be achieved?
4. How might the system knowledge be acquired, controlled and checked?

To answer the first question and attempt the second a system prototype was produced from a model of the diagnostic process (Fieschi, 1981; Fieschi *et al.*, 1982); from a critical study of the results obtained, the second version of the system is presented.

3.1   TESTING THE PROTOTYPE

This is based essentially on three concepts:

1. To place no restrictive hypothesis on the diagnoses, and in particular, to presuppose no exclusive diagnoses, thus bringing our model closer to clinical reality.
2. To activate various heuristics as a function of the symptomatology presented by the patient, that is, to define what will be called its 'context', and, after that, to resort to various rules chosen depending on the case.
3. To allow complete freedom for the deductive method to make logical step-wise progress through pursuit of signs which lead to the conclusion in a precise manner.

In fact, it is quite evident that the doctor does not always behave the same way throughout the search for a diagnosis. In the early days he listens to the patient describing his complaint without actively intervening to look for symptoms. At this stage he uses heuristics orientated knowledge which results from what is called the 'evocation power' of the recall-signs; that is, they use knowledge and approximate reasoning which can be modelled on the theory of fuzzy sets (Kaufmann, 1975), many valued logic (Rescher, 1969) or credibility functions (Shafer, 1976). We have applied SOULA's use of fuzzy logic (Soula, 1981) on the extended Modus Ponens and extended Modus Tollens (basic facts are given in Appendix 2) to many valued logic. This process merely plays a heuristic role which enables us to evoke some possible diagnostic channels. It will be necessary to explore these pathways logically for a second time through search for signs which will enable the final diagnosis to be established. This should be elaborated by a request for relevant complementary tests to identify the pathology. This reasoning sequence demonstrates the search for diagnostic certainty in medicine supported by unbiased, reliable knowledge. In the prototype beside the evocation knowledge, the system provides knowledge structured as a tree; with the sub-trees representing pathologies or different clinical forms of the same disease. The non-terminal nodes being group diagnoses whilst the terminal nodes gave aetiological diagnoses. Despite the development of heuristics of tree circuits based on the consequent nodes, on the frequency of 'success' attributed to each node, and on the in depth or saturation research strategies, the system behaviour does not give satisfaction in a good number of cases. In fact, the trees course with back-tracking did not allow for adjustment of patient data when necessary. Specifically, the interpretation of complementary tests was not considered as a whole but in terms of the node indicated; for example, if the system was trying to prove a myocardial infarct and the ECG did not support this diagnosis but presents an aspect on S1Q3, this vitally important information would not instigate, as one would wish it to, an immediate investigation of pulmonary embolism. At the same time, acceptable results of about 80% to 85% correct diagnoses recorded in the application of the system to epigastric pain have encouraged us to think that it is capable of reaching satisfactory expertise.

3.2   GENERAL PRESENTATION OF THE SYSTEM

The general plan is presented in Figure 3.1. The user communicates with the module MEDIUM ensuring coherent dialogue through his own knowledge (Joubert, 1981) and incorporating into the base signs and patient test results. Through a monitor, MEDIUM is connected with the decision module EXPERT, which carries out the tasks on its agenda using disease knowledge rules and rules of interpretation of complementary tests in accordance with the content of the data base. It may be said that whereas MEDIUM assures coherent dialogue, EXPERT ensures the relevance of the system discourse when in search of clinical signs or requesting para-clinical tests. This modular plan which separates the dialogue from the decision process has been investigated. It allows for separate development of the two phases, knowledge representations adapted to each problem and, above all, enables better demonstration and handling of the various levels arising during communication with the user. In fact, the knowledge base is divided to ensure consistent and

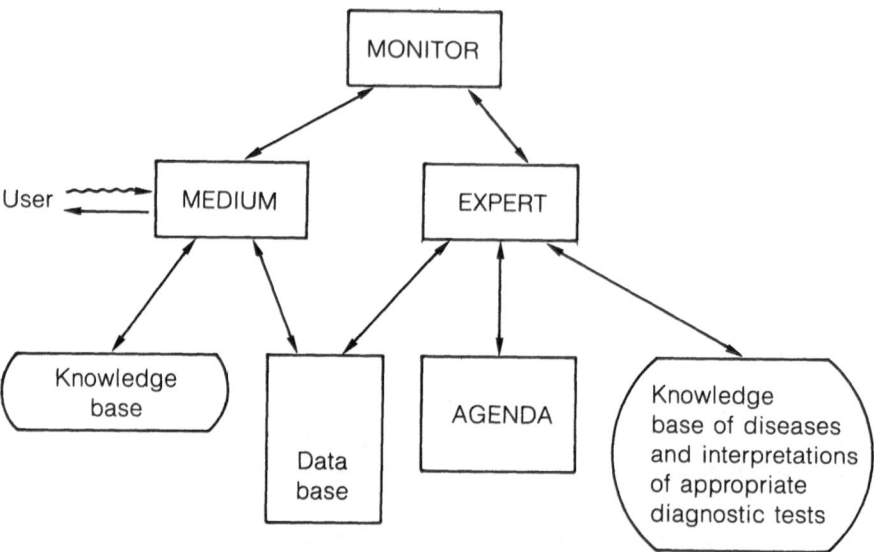

Fig. 3.1 General presentation of SPHINX. MEDIUM and EXPERT communicate through the MONITOR and together control the facts base which contains patient data and the conclusions of the EXPERT.

accurate data entry while the more typical medical knowledge is used to establish a diagnosis. For example, if the user tells the system that the patient is febrile then the dialogue module MEDIUM will make certain that he has not previously declared that the patient's temperature was normal; in addition, MEDIUM takes the initiative in asking the questions which characterize the fever better by asking how long has it lasted. If it has continued for several days how has it changed? What are the ranges of variation? Then applications such as looking for an asthenia or doing a blood count are also within the scope of the EXPERT module.

SPHINX has developed medical applications: one in the diagnosis of jaundice and the other an aid to diabetic therapy; examples are taken from each application.

3.3   ENTITIES FROM THE FIELD OF MEDICAL DISCOURSE

3.3.1   Definitions

Certain medical terms are called entities; they represent elementary facts in the medical sense or concepts in current practice such as symptoms, clinical signs, examination results, syndromes, diagnoses and therapies.

Each entity carries a name which can have synonyms, for example, pain, hurt, ache.

Before fully defining an entity the researcher characterizes it; for example, for a pain, he would specify its location, its extent, intensity and the circumstances which set it in motion. This set of attributes fully describe and qualify the entity.

Each attribute defines a semantic variable taking its values from a sub-group of the vocabulary. For example, the frequency of a symptom is a semantic variable which takes its values from the sub-vocabulary (never, rarely, often, always) that will be called semantic category (Joubert *et al.*, 1982a); it corresponds to a type of standard logic (Appendix 1). Definition of an entity by name and a list of attributes allows it to be represented symbolically in the language of a standard logic and thus to put it into an interpretation. An entity is represented in this language by an atom $P (X_1, X_2 \ldots X_n)$ where $X_1, X_2 \ldots X_n$ are values taken from the semantic categories $C_1, C_2 \ldots C_n$. So, when the system operator speaks of the entity P, the dialogue module, through a series of questions, he tries to find a way of substituting the variables X_i of the particle by constants belonging to various semantic categories C_i, to arrive at an expression of the entity in the form $P (a, b, c \ldots n)$, where $a \varepsilon C_1, b \varepsilon C_2 \ldots n \varepsilon C_n$. This entity represents an element of information about the patient, like a sign or a symptom which is assumed to be true; only this actual value will be taken into account.

Analysis of medical reasoning shows that the doctor in his rationale interprets quantitative data with scant reference to precise values except as a starting point. If, for example, the patient is a boy of 15 years, his exact age is of no real relevance to a diagnosis or therapy. The doctor will 'interpret' this information in the form: this is an adolescent. In the same way, if the patient has a temperature of 37.4°C the doctor conceives the temperature as normal. These considerations have led to representation of quantitative data by a value in the corresponding semantic category; and it is through this interpretation that the EXPERT module works.

3.3.2   Structuring of the semantic categories

The values of a semantic variable were regrouped into medically significant sub-groups. So, the entity APPETITE may be qualified by: 'Increased', 'Normal', 'Reduced', 'Greatly Increased', 'Slightly Increased', 'Greatly Reduced', 'Slightly Reduced'. The rationale of regrouping of qualities is consideration whether 'Greatly Increased' and 'Slightly Increased' are facts which accurately express the component 'Increased'.

The semantic category associated with the semantic variable 'change in appetite' is defined as a tree. Each named category is connected with

the root of the tree. The nodes which stem from the root define a primary level of division of the category. The concepts underlying these
nodes are mutually exclusive and describe the category completely; for
instance, one finds on the first level: Increased, Normal, Reduced. The
nodes which stem from the first level define a second level which
contributes a degree of supplementary detail by reference to the level
above. Below the node 'Increased' will be found 'Greatly Increased' and
'Slightly Increased'; the 'Normal' node will have no descendant; and the
nodes 'Greatly Reduced' and 'Slightly Reduced' will be linked to
'Reduced'. Division at each level for each section is exclusive. A temperature cannot at the same time be increased and normal; if it is
increased it will be slightly raised or greatly increased but in no circumstances could it be both.

A semantic category has a tree structure whose leaves or terminal
nodes express full details of the information.

Examples of semantic categories:

TEMPERATURE is qualified by a 'MODIFICATION' attribute:

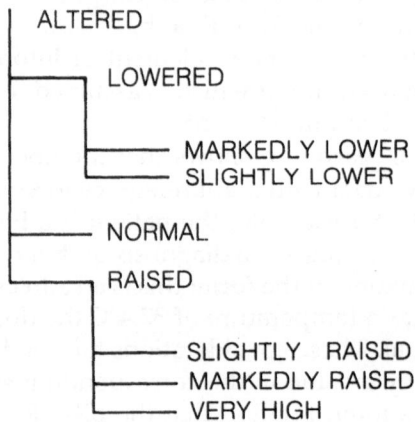

The sign VOMITING is characterized by 'PRESENCE' and 'CIRCUM-
STANCES':

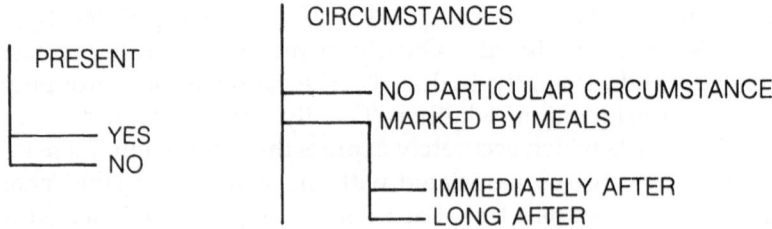

This representation unites quantitative and qualitative data and subsequently enables the EXPERT module to process it purely with symbols.

3.3.3 The specimens

These were introduced to allow the user a more concise, more accurate and better technical expression. For each entity it is possible to attach one or more specimens which frame a means of access to this entity. For example, the operator has a choice when conveying information about his patient's temperature between the expressions:

TEMPERATURE OF 39.2°C
TEMPERATURE GREATLY INCREASED
HIGH FEVER

The first two expressions refer to TEMPERATURE explicitly. The third uses the word 'FEVER' which is a specimen of the entity TEMPERATURE; that is, beside the fact that FEVER refers to the same concept expressed by TEMPERATURE it specifies that it is 'RAISED'. Thus the specimens provide information and certain attributes; they are a form of partial achievement of an entity.

Examples:

TACHYCARDIA would be expressed by	PULSE (raised)
MAN	SEX (male), AGE (adult)
ANOREXIA	APPETITE (greatly reduced)
FEBRILE	TEMPERATURE (slightly raised)

3.3.4 Entity classes

The advantage of defining classes of entities is especially obvious when one refers to them for interpretation of a test. These signs are never looked for alone or requested in isolation; for example, the number of red cells, of leucocytes, basophils, neutrophils, eosinophils, lymphocytes, monocytes and reticulocytes, belong to this category; they are grouped as the Formula Count. A class of entities is a tree-structured framework with the entity defining the class linked to the root of this tree, and a sub-class entity is linked to an underlying node.

Example:
X-ray of the thorax: the postero-anterior view is explained with the aid of the entity structuring which follows.

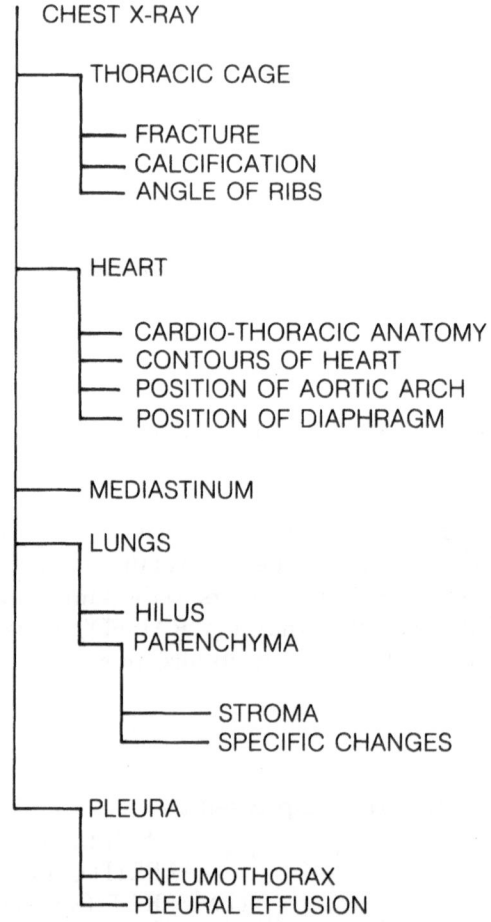

3.3.5 Principles of structuring of the facts base

The entities are recorded sequentially in the fact base. It includes the whole attribute called 'CONDITION' which enables the entity to be placed in the development of the disease and, on the other hand, to know whether this entity states a clinical fact, or information from the questioning, the result of a paraclinical examination, or even an established diagnosis. CONDITION is also tree-structured and presented in the following form:

It should be emphasized that the coding of this attribute conforms to the order:

Clinical sign < Examination sign < Paraclinical result

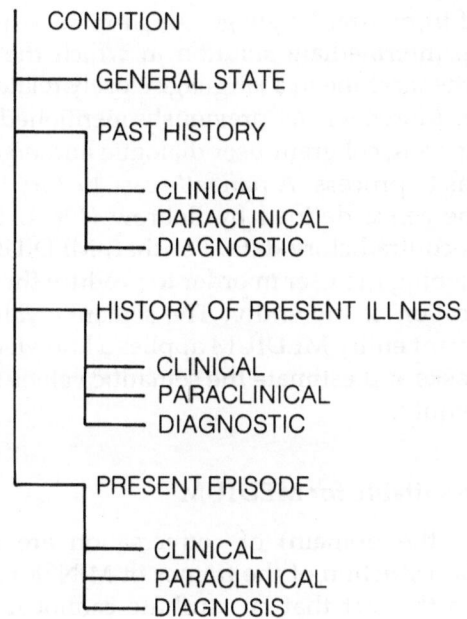

```
CONDITION
 ├── GENERAL STATE
 ├── PAST HISTORY
 │    ├── CLINICAL
 │    ├── PARACLINICAL
 │    └── DIAGNOSTIC
 ├── HISTORY OF PRESENT ILLNESS
 │    ├── CLINICAL
 │    ├── PARACLINICAL
 │    └── DIAGNOSTIC
 └── PRESENT EPISODE
      ├── CLINICAL
      ├── PARACLINICAL
      └── DIAGNOSIS
```

The significance of this observation will become clear when the system control is discussed.

Entities expressing age, sex and height, etc., are allocated implicitly to the condition: FACT OF GENERAL CATEGORY. Former diagnoses and former surgical operations are in 'ANTECEDENT', the warning signs which motivate the consultation in 'DISEASE HISTORY' and the clinical examination results in 'PRESENT EPISODE'. Two products of a single entity may be found in two different 'conditions'; for example, surgical operation in the antecedents and patient actually post-operative. MEDIUM in the course of the dialogue fixes the value of this particular attribute which enables structuring of the data base and plays roughly the same role as the contexts tree of MYCIN or EMYCIN. That is, it allows amalgamations of entities to operate along with certain processes of the data base: the print-out of the contents of the data base, which can be asked for at any time (for example), is done by amalgamating relative entities in an identical situation. The attribute situation frames the clinical problem and in this way leads to better control.

3.4   PRODUCTION AND USE OF THE ENTITIES IN THE DIALOGUE, MEDIUM (JOUBERT, 1981)

The dialogue module was developed to avoid the operator having to express himself in an restricted artificial language, without allowing him to express himself in natural language. As in many expert systems we have opted for an intermediate solution in which the module allows interchange with the machine in a language closely related to the routine medical discourse. Moreover, as previously mentioned this module is responsible for ensuring coherent user dialogue and no contradiction in the data that he has to process. A patient's case history thus makes up a coherent set in the sense defined by Bobrow (1968), that is, a set of complete and non-contradictory data. For that, MEDIUM may take the initiative by questioning the user in order to produce the necessary components for application of the entity. The semantic values of the attributes for each relevant entity MEDIUM applies a knowledge appropriate to perform these tasks and estimate the semantic values of the attributes for each relevant entity.

3.4.1 Knowledge suitable for MEDIUM

The entities (from the domain) of conversation are represented by frames which are a restriction of the frames of MINSKY. This limitation rests essentially on the fact that an attribute cannot itself be a frame. Each attribute becomes a slot of the frame entity and it may be necessary to fill up this slot to refer to other entities. So, for example, evaluation of the attribute for interpreting the number of red blood cells must take account of two entities, AGE and SEX; MEDIUM sets up for this purpose a knowledge which is given below (entities are presented in capitals, attribute values in lower case and the numerical value in italics:

NUMBER OF RED CELLS (RC):

IF (RC ≥ 4.5 AND RC ≤ 6) AND (AGE = adolescent OR AGE = adult)
    AND (SEX = male)
  OR (RC ≥ 4 AND RC ≤ 5.5) AND
    (AGE = adolescent OR AGE = adult) AND (Sex = female))
  OR ((RC ≥ 4 AND RC ≤ 5.5) AND
    (AGE = infant OR AGE = young child))
  OR ((RC ≥ 4 AND RC ≤ 6) AND (AGE = newborn))
THEN NB RC = normal
IF ((RC > 6) AND (AGE = adolescent OR AGE = adult) AND
    (SEX = male))
  OR ((RC > 5.5) and (AGE = adolescent OR AGE = adult) AND
    (SEX = female))
  OR ((RC > 5.5) AND (AGE = infant OR AGE = young child))
  OR ((RC > 6) AND (AGE = new born))
THEN NB RC = increased

It may be necessary to refer to other entities to evaluate an attribute, as in the preceding case, or more commonly to abide by the prevailing commonsense opinion. For example, if a patient complains of 'digestive problems' the system might take an interest in the dietary habits of the subject asking if he consumes alcohol and how much? if the subject is on a diet, whether he often eats too much at mealtimes. A slot may be defined by a schema which explains the production terms of the entity. For example:

The entity PREGNANT WOMAN is subject to a production condition:
(AGE = adolescent OR AGE = young adult) AND (SEX = female)

This condition forms a slot in the schema which ensures consistent user dialogue, but it is quite likely that these relative conditions represent further medical constraints and lead to sanction of complementary tests while bearing contra-indication in mind; for example, the entity HEPATIC NEEDLE BIOPSY is subject to the condition:

(PROTHROMBIN LEVEL = normal OR slightly decreased)

This condition leads the system to ask for a prothrombin level (TP) and to be sure that it is normal or subnormal before requesting a hepatic needle biopsy which is contra-indicated in the case where the TP is greatly reduced.

A further example: ASCITES TAP is subject to the condition:

(ASCITE = sufficiently important)

which declares that only a sufficiently important effusion will be tappable.

In MEDIUM-permissible dialogue the user provides data to the system on one entity at a time; thus one may provide data which allows assessment of attributes in two ways:

1. Either by direct association of the attribute with the entity, e.g. FREQUENT VOMITING FOR A WEEK
2. Or by engaging in brief dialogue with the user each time that he provides insufficient data to fill the slots of the corresponding frame.

Example: user: VOMITING
         MEDIUM: is it frequent?
         user: YES
         MEDIUM: for how long?
         user: FOR A WEEK

When the data normally expected are quantitative they are expressed in 'semantic values', as shown in the example below, which gives an idea of connection between procedures and definitions of the entities. The procedures are specific for those attributes to which they are linked. Each attribute is associated with a questionnaire whose development fits the condition and the replies already received. The replies allow the attribute to be assigned to one of the values of the semantic category.

Example

Condition of evaluation of the attribute 'estimation' of the entity temperature. t is the numerical value given by the user:

IF $(t > 36.4)$ AND $(t < 37.7)$ THEN normal
IF $(t > 37.7)$ THEN raised
IF $(t > 37.7)$ AND $(t < 38.5)$ THEN slightly raised
IF $(t > 38.5)$ AND $(t < 39.5)$ THEN greatly raised
IF $(t > 39.5)$ THEN very greatly raised
IF $(t < 36.4)$ THEN lowered
IF $(t < 36.4)$ THEN slightly lowered
IF $(t < 35.6)$ THEN very low

3.4.2 Consistency of data in the facts base

MEDIUM is designed to ensure consistency in the two following cases:

1. When the datum itself is inconsistent detection is then straightforward; for example, where a value is outside the minimum and maximum limits, such as: AGE = 120 YEARS, RED BLOOD CELLS = 100 MILLIONS. In such cases the system repeats the question until a plausible value is obtained.
2. When the datum contradicts the information in the facts base; for example, the data base contains: AGE = adolescent, SEX = female; and the user provides the following information: ONE YEAR AFTER MENOPAUSE. This type of difficulty is dealt with by ignoring the entity which introduced the contradiction and is therefore not acceptable. If a datum is reported on the genital tract of a patient without specifying his age the system finds it impossible to state positively whether the data are consistent or incoherent. It will seek to specify the patient's age before accepting or refusing the information.

3.4.3 Structure of the facts base

The facts base is developed by incorporation of the entities as and when they are produced. MEDIUM initiates sequential entry of n-tuplets which describe the entities. They have the following structure:

⟨name of the entity⟩ (⟨condition attribute⟩, ⟨attribute 1⟩, ...,
⟨attribute⟩ R)

The condition attribute is as specified earlier, a structuring component of the data base. Just as there are multivalent parameters in MYCIN, SPHINX is able to define entities which may be present in several forms concomitantly in the same condition; for example, a patient may complain of several pains which are not mutually exclusive, such as headaches and epigastric pain. The system recognizes these entities and as soon as it acquires one tries to ensure that it is unique to the patient; for example, if a cervical adenopathy is reported the system will request a search of all the ganglion surfaces for a possible adenopathy. In addition, MEDIUM provides a knowledge which is able to process inconsistencies within multiple entities; thus, in this way, it would refuse to enter two complaints both situated in the right hypochondrium of which the first was very severe whereas the second was quite weak.

3.5 EXPERT: ORGANIZATION AND USE OF THE KNOWLEDGE

Expert knowledge is mainly expressed in the form of production rules operating through n-uplets which are the entities from the domain of medical language. They are of the form:

IF premises THEN effects

Each premise is a combination of entities expressing a condition for production of the actions represented in the rule.

The consultation begins by activation of the EVOCATION rules which initiates an agenda of goals to weigh; for each objective the system then uses a goal-directed control structure. However, where a data directed approach is needed to make use of a small number of estimations provided at a given time, such as results of paraclinical investigations, SPHINX proposes ways of modifying the agenda and thereby exerting a control over user behaviour.

3.5.1 Contexts

Definition

The model presenting a system aid to medical decision-making is goal-directed and exhaustively considers all the possible diagnoses that are unacceptable for a number of reasons. The main ones are:

1. Such a system does not take sufficiently into account those facts in the data base which cause it to respond in a simplistic and rather unintelligent way.
2. Such a strategy cannot be seriously proposed if the medical application bears upon numerous possible diagnoses and therefore, a large number of rules.

An heuristic process was therefore created which limits the maximum number of acceptable hypotheses and ignores those patient's signs which are not relevant. Alternatively, it identifies a datum which is important for the follow-up investigations. So 'coarse grain' knowledge (Aikins, 1980) was specified in contrast to 'fine grain' knowledge in the rules. This distinction allows the control structure to use 'coarse grain' knowledge to determine the general context of the patient; that is, the list of diagnostic hypotheses which should be considered before looking for more specific data to affirm or reject each one. The hypotheses are developed by reference to a number of 'clinical frameworks' and the

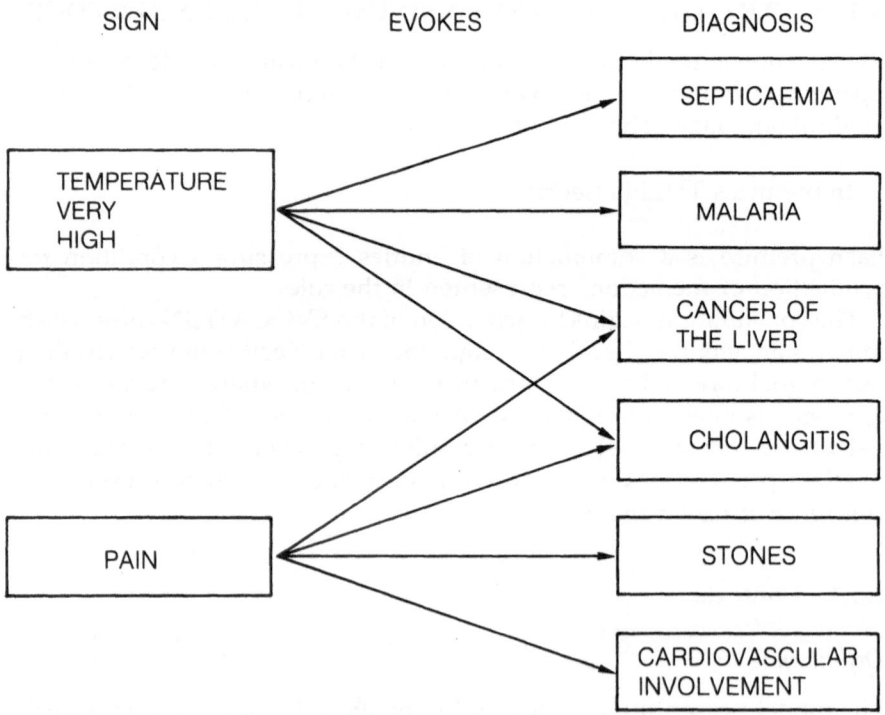

Fig. 3.2

choice of context for a given patient is made by estimating the most probable framework; this constitutes the initial phase of expert reasoning. A context is defined by reference to the data, entities and circumstances which should be considered when describing the condition in which a list of diagnostic routes be entered on the agenda. As a result, the rules represent a highly specialized knowledge which enable formal diagnosis to be made while prior to that the system will use a knowledge which calls on weighted assertions to prescribe the patient's context. One of the first problems that had to be solved when representing the system knowledge was how to assist the expert to construct the intended diagnostic domain so as to lead him to define various contexts; in other words, the clinical frameworks typified by definite symptoms and the diagnoses to be derived from them. Figures 3.2 and 3.3 are schematic examples of the concept of context.

Definition of contexts involves the following operation:
   These contexts are mainly characterized by general signs of great importance to diagnostic orientation and by recall signs; knowing whether

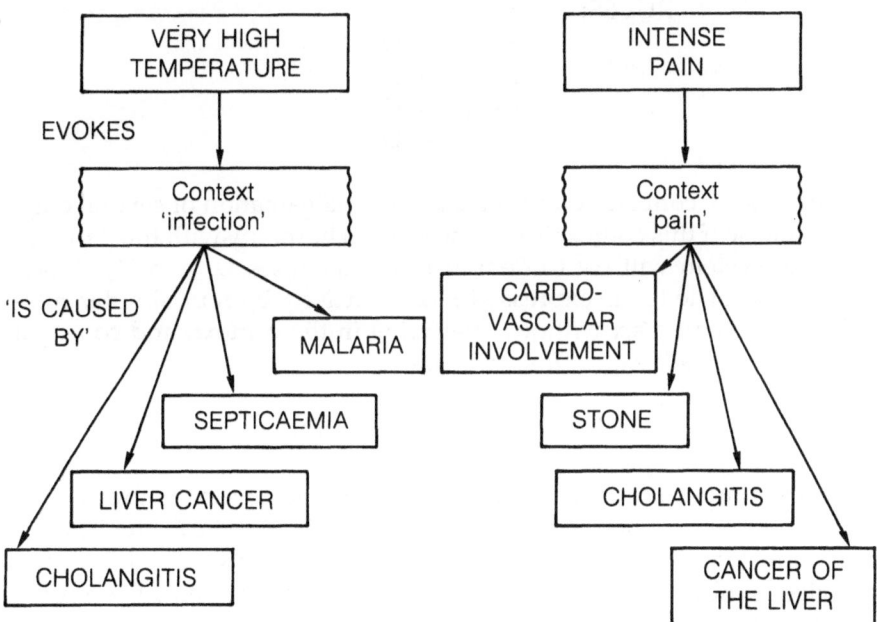

Fig. 3.3 Schematic concept of context. The contexts are Pople's 'intermediary pathological markers'. They enable the symptomatology of the patient to be characterized and managed.

a patient was admitted to hospital urgently or came by appointment, whether he is 3 or 58 years old, whether he has behavioural problems or not, are facts which have a definite diagnosis evoking power.

The acquisition of this knowledge allows the contexts to be deferred and affects the writing of the 'close grained' rules; it limits the proliferation of rules, many of which would be proved useless. To specify the concept of these contexts the following six knowledge rules lead to diagnoses D_1 and D_2:

$$R_1: \quad A \wedge B \rightarrow D_1$$
$$R_2: (A \vee C) \wedge E \rightarrow D_1$$
$$R_3: \quad C \wedge B \rightarrow D_1$$
$$R_4: \quad C \wedge H \rightarrow D_2$$
$$R_5: \quad A \wedge H \rightarrow D_2$$
$$R_6: (C \vee A) \wedge F \rightarrow D_2$$

The diagnoses D_1 and D_2 will be regrouped under a context characterized by the signs A and C; so the knowledge will be in the form:

Context: the patient presents A or C
RULES:

$$R_1': B \rightarrow D_1$$
$$R_2': E \rightarrow D_1$$
$$R_3': F \rightarrow D_2$$
$$R_4': H \rightarrow D_2$$

This process of context definition leads to amalgamation of several diagnoses, and so if this context is the one most in harmony with the patient's case, the system will try to demonstrate diagnoses D_1 and D_2. Moreover, the knowledge is expressed more concisely by four simpler rules than the preceding six without interfering in the context, and could for that matter be reduced to just two rules:

$$B \vee E \rightarrow D_1 \text{ and } F \vee H \rightarrow D_2$$

Another important concept represented by the context is the expression of imprecise knowledge which is found in medical literature in such forms as: 'the causes of the jaundice will be investigated: a pre-jaundice syndrome suggests hepatitis: pseudo-influenzal episode, digestive disorders, migraines, pruritis the previous week; a marked change in general condition with significant loss of weight, anorexia, debility suggesting a neoplasic cause', or again: 'pruritis and bradycardia point to an intra-hepatic or extra-hepatic cholestasis; discovery of an anaemia and dystrophy suggests an haemolytic jaundice; neuro-psychic disorders with change in personality are evidence of an hepatic encephalopathy'.

Jaundice-related diagnoses have therefore been amalgamated into nine contexts, such as the hepatic encephalopathy or the cholestasis context. In the encephalopathy context, for example, will be found diagnoses of cirrhosis, cancer of the liver, certain types of hepatitis, alcoholism and acute steatosis of pregnancy. This context is characterized by presence of neuro-psychic problems, flapping tremor and personality change. Presentation of one or several of these signs strongly supports the context whereas their absence rejects it. It could be said that these signs are not specific to one diagnosis but to a group of diagnoses; they thereby characterize the context. Moreover, these signs are sufficiently sensitive for their simultaneous absence to direct rejection of the search for the diagnostic links of this context. The result is that the user and the clinical investigation determine the diagnosis which is established with the aid of tests. Certain pinpoint signs, mainly recall signs, will be empowered exclusively to evoke or reject the various contexts. The composition of evocation and rejection powers for signs presented by the patient leads to choice of the context; that is, through those diagnostic routes that the system will follow to confirm one or several of them by a fuzzy inference mechanism which will be explained later on.

A certain analogy carr be made between, on the one hand, our contexts of amalgamated diagnoses and the CENTAUR prototypes, and, on the other, the knowledge of the evocation and rejection powers and the triggering rules of this system.

Knowledge which refers to the contexts

Each context is defined as a set of diagnoses known to the system. The choice of context is made at the consultation during evocation phase which is set in motion as soon as the system has enough knowledge to consider it pertinent; for which, EXPERT uses a knowledge of the type:

$$A \text{ evokes (weighting } = e) \ C \ (1)$$
$$\neg A \text{ rejects (weighting } = r) \ C \ (2)$$

where A is the expression of a typical entity with evoking power e for context C, and (2) conveys context C in the absence of A rejects with a weighting r. Evocation and rejection capacities are set empirically by the expert with values between 0 and 1.

Example:

DEBILITY	(Recent, severe)	EVOKES (0.4) CTXT CHANGE IN GENERAL STATE
DEBILITY	(Recent, severe)	REJECTS (0.3) CTXT CHANGE IN GENERAL STATE
TEMPERATURE	(Greatly raised)	EVOKES (0.7) CTXT INFECTIOUS
TEMPERATURE	(Raised)	EVOKES (0.4) CTXT PAINFUL
TEMPERATURE	(Greatly raised)	REJECTS (0.7) CTXT INFECTIOUS
N.B. DEBILITY	(Recent, intense)	REJECTS (0.3) CTXT CHANGE IN GENERAL STATE

should be interpreted as: *absence* of a recent and severe debility rejects the context of change in general state with a force 0.3. Only the knowledge used in the evocation phase leads to an approximate reasoning.

3.5.2 Production rules

SPHINX rules are of classical form: IF cause THEN effects. Each cause is an entity conjunction; an effect may be development of the data base or of the agenda. After introduction of the syntax of the system rules, four types of SPHINX rules are presented: evocation rules, rules of diagnostic knowledge, rules of examination interpretation and rules of conflict resolution. They have the same general form but differ in their use.

Syntax of the SPHINX rules

(An asterix * indicates that the material in brackets may be repeated one or more times.)

Rule	= IF	cause	THEN	effect		
premise	= condition	condition	AND	condition	*	
effect	= conclusion	conclusion	AND	conclusion	*	
condition	= entity	entity	AND	condition	*	
conclusion	= entity verb entity	*	entity	AND	conclusion	*
verb	= TO ASK FOR	TO LOOK FOR	TO THINK OF			
	TO IGNORE	TO EVOKE	TO TRIGGER			
	TO PRESCRIBE	TO ALTER				
	= clinical sign	paraclinical sign	syndrome			
	interpretation of examination	therapy	context			

Evocation rules

These are rules triggered in forward chaining which are of the form:

IF ALTERED BEHAVIOUR AND CONFUSION THEN TO EVOKE
(CTXT ENCEPHALOPATHY)

IF CHILD AND SLIGHT JAUNDICE AND PALLOR THEN TO
  EVOKE (CTXT CONGENITAL ANAEMIA)
IF PAIN AND PALE STOOLS THEN TO EVOKE (CTXT PAIN-
  FUL)
IF MEDICINAL TRT THEN TO EVOKE (CTXT IATROGENIC)

There are seventeen of these rules applied to jaundice. They play the
part of the triggering rules of CENTAUR or PIP.

At initiation the system agenda requires that the task of evocation be
carried out for which the user will use the evocation rules in the order in
which they appear. The first rule triggered allows evocation to proceed
which is completed with development of the agenda where diagnoses
that the system will attempt to substantiate. In the case where the data
base provided spontaneously by the consultant is inadequate, the rules
lead to context definition asking for further information such as the
patient's age, his state of mind, or the need for urgent (hospital)
admission.

Diagnostic or therapeutic knowledge rules

These rules enable diagnoses to be worked out or therapies proposed.
The system considers them according to the goal so they are triggered in
reverse chaining, which is a classical process of step-by-step decomposition of the initial problem into better defined sub-aims. The 'cause'
part of a rule is a combination of entities which must agree with the data
input on any given patient so that precise 'effects' can be guaranteed
in the rule. Some examples of diagnostic knowledge rules applied to
jaundice are the following:

R5 IF: Bilirubin mainly conjugated
              Blood count suggests infection
              Sedimentation rate is slightly increased
              Murphy's sign positive
THEN: Cholangitis suspected
R72 IF:

              Cholangitis suspected
              Common bile duct lithiasis on echotomography of
                the bile ducts
THEN:

              Cholangitis
R6 IF:

              Cholangitis suspected
              Echotomography of the bile ducts: total dilatation
                of the common bile duct

	Calculus present in the ampulla of Vater on retrograde catherization of the papilla
THEN:	
	Cholangitis
R20 IF:	
	Cancer of the liver suspected
	Image of metastases on liver echotomography
THEN:	
	Secondary cancer of the liver
TO THINK OF:	Cancer of the pancreas, cancer of the bile ducts, cancer of the ampulla of Vater, cancer of the gall bladder
TO ASK FOR:	echotomography of the pancreas, fibroscopy
TO IGNORE:	cholangitis, abscess of the liver, hepatitis, malaria, septicaemia.

The reverse chaining is produced from the high level of the goal, diagnostic or therapeutic, to the clinical data of the low level. Following input of the rules the system locates the objectives and the sub-objectives and lists each corresponding rule. The input order of rules is quite arbitrary, which is one advantage of this representation. For each rule the user evaluates the cause: if one of these entities contradicts the data base the rule is suppressed and its 'effects' are not undertaken. If there is a cause entity missing from the data base (apart from an objective or sub-objective) the system is unable to deduce EXPERT questions MEDIUM to obtain the necessary information. If the user cannot reply, the information remains unknown and the rule is in check. The general inference procedure corresponds to a depth-first exploration of an AND/OR tree; each node AND corresponds to the premise of a rule, the OR nodes outlining the various rules which prescribe the objective or sub-objectives. The knowledge rules do not carry weighting. They lead to definite conclusions; therefore, as soon as an objective is reached through one rule there is no further need to try other related rules. There are problems set by this resolution strategy which will be discussed.

Examination interpretation rules

Some entities are amalgamated into classes (section 3.3.4) and should be read in the aggregate; particularly in the case of paraclinical examinations whose general interpretation develops from elementary descriptive entities. This knowledge is expressed in the form of antecedent production rules, that is, triggered in forward chaining which takes into account all the components which the examination reveals, rather than a limited interpretation within the framework of the system objective. The use of such verbs as TO THINK OF, TO LOOK FOR, TO IGNORE, which will be referred to again later, provide a system which is data directed not only in the initial phase of the consultation but also when paraclinical results are interpreted. They permit update in the agenda contents and in the user dialogue to keep pace with the patient symptoms presented:

Examples:

R8 IF:
>   White cell count raised
>   Neutrophil fraction increased

THEN:
>   Blood count infection

R2 IF:
>   Haemoglobin low
>   Red cells increased
>   Microcytosis
>   Hypochromia

THEN:
>   Pseudo microcytic polycythaemia (polyglobulism)
>   TO IGNORE: Addison Biermer anaemia
>   TO THINK OF: Haemoglobinopathy

R7 IF:
>   Haemoglobin low
>   Normochromia
>   Macrocytosis

THEN:
>   Normochromic macrocytic anaemia
>   TO THINK OF: Addison Biermer anaemia, cirrhosis

R17 IF:
>   Haemoglobin low
>   MCV low
>   Microcytosis

THEN:
>   Iron-deficiency anaemia
>   TO IGNORE: Addison Biermer anaemia

Rules of conflict resolution

SPHINX uses four rules to represent its general strategy for conflict resolution. They are triggered in forward chaining and expressed in the following way:

1. IF EVALUATION (Rule, TRUE) THEN TO TRIGGER (Rule)
2. IF EVALUATION (Rule, FALSE) THEN TO ELIMINATE (Rule)
3. IF LIST (Empty) THEN DEMONSTRATION (goal, CHECK) AND TO CHANGE (goal)
4. IF LIST (Not empty) THEN TO DIRECT AND DEMONSTRATION (goal, to start)

A rule must be chosen from a list and against each choice rules 1. and 2. are tested. If the data base considers the premise of the chosen rule to be TRUE it is triggered and the goal is then reached; if the data base is equipped to affirm that the rule under examination may not be triggered, the rule is eliminated from the conflict list. These two rules are applied in two cases: if the list is empty through elimination of all the rules, then rule 3. is applied; if the list is not empty it will be processed by rule 4. Rule 3. confirms that the goal is in check if the list of elected rules is empty; the objective is abandoned and the user moves on to the next goal. If the list is not empty, rule 4. recalls the TO COMMAND procedure and returns to the goal demonstration. Rules are classified according to the entities which they contain. The rule chosen is the one calling on the minimum number of paraclinical facts. This heuristic choice is made to maintain coherence of the discourse for which it is better to request clinical data before paraclinical entities. In addition, this choice has the benefit of reducing research costs.

These four reasoning rules are comparable to the meta-rules used in TEIRESIAS (Davis, 1980a) or to those proposed by EMYCIN (Van Melle, 1980), in that they encode a strategic knowledge for the reverse chaining control of the rules by dynamic reorganization of the list of candidate rules. It is well worth noting that these meta-rules do not alter the system knowledge in the domain, they represent a knowledge which leads to greater efficiency in the search for signs and the demand for tests.

3.5.3 Inference mechanisms

Mechanisms are presented which allow deductions to be made by SPHINX. The resolution of the data in the data base and the rules premises are considered successively, then the mechanism leading to fuzzy reasoning for the choice of patient context.

SPHINX matching

The process reduces two literals to a singleton (cf. Appendix 1). In its generally recognized meaning this process can be practised on literals containing variables which can be substituted by terms to make the literals identical. It can sometimes be ranked as 'pattern matching' but it is less limited in its application. 'Pattern matching' does not usually allow appearance of variables in both the expressions submitted to 'matching'; in fact, an expression 'goal' is applied which may be super-imposed on an expression 'fact', which makes the 'pattern matching' process non-symmetrical.

The SPHINX entities are clearly manifest as literals of typed logic in which each attribute takes its values from a form determined by its position in the literal. Knowledge is represented by symbolic trees terminating in nodes to which are attached terms without variables, giving a degree of precision crossing from root to leaves. The organization shown within the categories may be represented by the term DEPENDANT OF which is comparable to the expressions ELEMENT-OF and IS-A (Joubert, 1982b).

The term DEPENDANT-OF is defined in all the semantic categories; its properties are presented in the following principles:

If C is a semantic category and R a related symbol n-ary defined by $C_1 \times C_2 \times \ldots \times C_n$

$$F_0 = \forall C \, \forall X \in C \qquad \text{DEPENDANT-OF}(X, X)$$

$$F_1 = \forall X_1 \in C_1 \, \forall X_2 \in C_2 \ldots X_n \in C_n$$

$$\forall y_1 \in C_1 \, \forall y_2 \in C_2 \qquad y_n \in C_n$$

$$\text{DEPENDANT-OF}(x_1, y_1) \wedge \ldots \wedge \text{DEPENDANT-OF}(X_n, y_n) \wedge R(X_1, \ldots X_n)$$
$$\rightarrow R(y_1, \ldots y_n)$$

These principles are comparable to those of the equality in the case of the terms. The example following demonstrates the properties of the term DEPENDANT-OF:

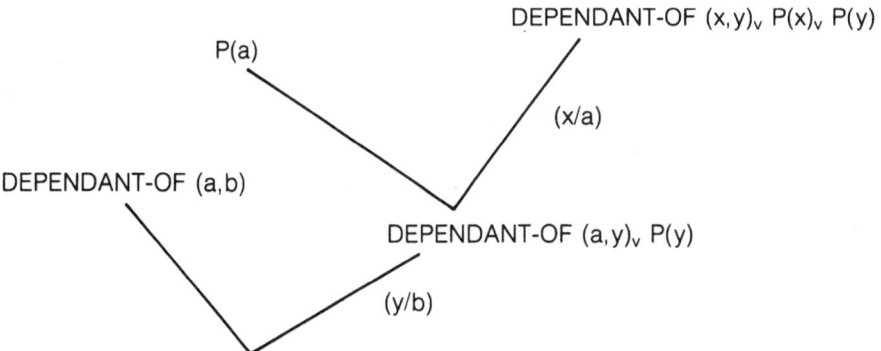

If a and b are constants where DEPENDANT-OF (a, b) is satisfied in an interpretation I; if P(a) is complied with in I then so is P(b).

Where terms comply with an element in the category they comply also with its ascendants. Conversely, besides the terms that they satisfy themselves, elements of a category may only comply with their ascendant terms.

For the sake of reducing the number of successive resolutions and to reduce the response time the term DEPENDANT-OF was included in the matching process. The tree structure of the categories incorporates a special coding which avoids having to detail all the element pairs in the data base which satisfy the term DEPENDANT-OF. The user is skilled and takes responsibility for the use of the two principles F_0 and F_1. Matching in SPHINX therefore takes into account both the structure and the properties of the semantic classifications to increase user efficiency.

Example:

Consider the category giving the variation in sedimentation rate (E.S.R.).

Reduced (↓)
    Markedly reduced (↓↓)

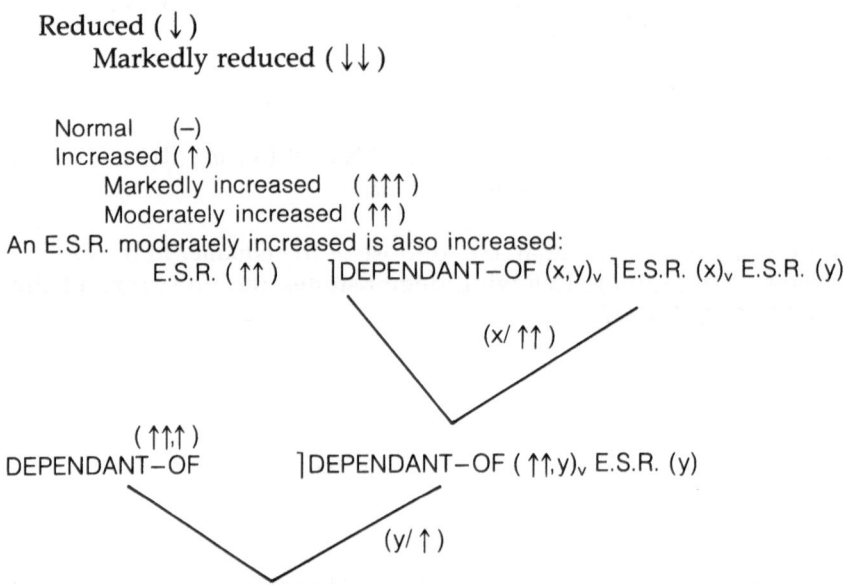

Normal   (−)
Increased (↑)
        Markedly increased   (↑↑↑)
        Moderately increased (↑↑)
An E.S.R. moderately increased is also increased:
                E.S.R. (↑↑)   ]DEPENDANT−OF (x,y)$_v$]E.S.R. (x)$_v$ E.S.R. (y)

                                        (x/ ↑↑)

            (↑↑↑)
DEPENDANT−OF   ]DEPENDANT−OF (↑↑,y)$_v$ E.S.R. (y)

                                (y/ ↑)

            E.S.R. (↑)

Suppose that the data base and knowledge base are made up in the following way:

Data base	*Knowledge base*

⋮
Bilirubin mainly conjugated
Blood count infection
E.S.R. moderately increased
MURPHY's sign
⋮
	⋮
	IF Bilirubin mainly conjugated
	          E.S.R. increased
	          Blood count infection
	          MURPHY's sign
	THEN
	          Suspected cholangitis
	⋮

Matching could be carried out on the E.S.R. just as on the other entities and suspected cholangitis will be added to the data base.

It must be emphasized that representation of the entities in SPHINX allows the calculation of the predicates and inferences to be made. This distinguishes it from other known expert systems which are currently operational in medicine and which work generally in propositional logic weighted by credibility factors.

Evocation and rejection

It appears that the majority of complex problems cannot be solved by a small set of pre-defined rules applied in an all or nothing manner, and applies equally to the intricate problem of choosing a diagnostic route. Therefore, to identify the context or contexts closest to the clinical picture a fuzzy 'pattern matching' module was created which can be activated by the evocation rules and is activated for a given patient by the first rule triggered.

This 'fuzzy pattern matching' module is used once only during the consultation to initiate the agenda by a number of hypotheses.

Each context is defined by the entity prototypes which are allocated weightings, allowing calculation of the context evocation force by the prototype. This empirical knowledge provided by the expert leads to operation of the evocation heuristic.

We were drawn by Zadeh's theory of reasoning (Zadeh, 1979) as well as the work of Soula (1981) to produce an evocation reasoning. The general schema for deduction of the conventional Modus Ponens follows:

$$
\begin{array}{ll}
\text{Knowledge} \\
\text{rules}
\end{array}
\left[
\begin{array}{l}
X \text{ is } A^1 \\
\text{IF } X \text{ is } A^1 \text{ THEN } Y \text{ is } B_1 \text{ Rule } R_1 \\
\text{IF } X \text{ is } A_2 \text{ THEN } Y \text{ is } B_2 \text{ Rule } R_2 \\
\cdots\cdots\cdots\cdots\cdots\cdots\cdots\cdots \\
\underline{\text{IF } X \text{ is } A_n \text{ THEN } Y \text{ is } B_n \text{ Rule } R_n}
\end{array}
\right.
$$

Conclusion: Y is B^1

The knowledge which leads to the inference is made up of the rules R_i. The problem is to identify to what extent the observation A^1 confirms that Y is B^1 from the rules R_i. $A_i \ldots A_n$, $B_1 \ldots B_n$, B^1 are in this case fuzzy sets in the language fields U (for $A_1 \ldots A_n$, A^1) and V (for $B_1 \ldots B_n$, B^1) (Cayrol, 1980). Various processes have been proposed for this kind of approximate reasoning including Zadeh (1975), Soula (1981), Mizumoto *et al.* (1979) and Tsukamoto (1979); but all are produced from numerical variables (e.g. age or temperature) although in the general expression it may be any field whatever. In fact, a numerical language field more readily defines a fuzzy set by a membership function. In our experience the main difficulty is with the entities (our atomic formulae) whose attributes take their value from purely linguistic language fields. For example, the entity 'appetite' has an attribute which can take values in the following semantic category in which it is very difficult to introduce a numerical language to quantify the resemblance of two elements of the semantic category.

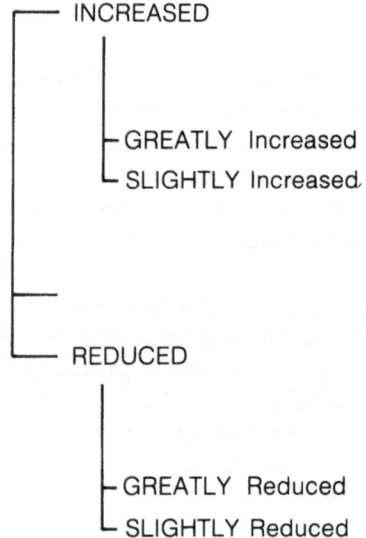

Some authors (Zadeh, 1975; Sanchez, 1979) consider INCREASED, NORMAL as fuzzy linguistic variables where GREATLY increased, SLIGHTLY increased, are values of these variables and are defined as fuzzy sets. The operation of these concepts requires the user to work out the appetite property of the patient from the set. Similar techniques are proposed in various other expert systems; in MYCIN it is possible to give an assertion with a credibility coefficient, for example, the system can be told that the patient is exposed to the risk of contact with a given germ, with a credibility 0.8. The approach set out below was preferred for the following reasons:

1. Expression in a numerically weighted way of what one feels, such as pains, or of what one concludes, like diminished appetite, is not natural. It seems inevitable to introduce a 'false' quantification on the one hand because — and it has been shown in studies — such judgements are not made as a continuous segment but rather on a scale of 3 to 5 values; and on the other hand, because the concept of 'increased' or 'reduced' is naturally linguistically fuzzy, it is very difficult to appraise the meaning of the user's weighting coefficient.
2. The credibility given by the user is not necessarily in keeping with the way that the expert weighted the rule or the knowledge.

Ways have therefore been sought to allow the operator to use directly his natural vocabulary. This vocabulary is constructed like a tree in the semantic category and it is on the basis of this structure that we envisaged estimating to what extent 'greatly increased' could be replaced by 'increased', in an evocation knowledge to give a degree of semantic conformity between two elements (of the tree). It is machine calculated by an algorithm of which the expert may be aware so that he can take account of it when constructing the semantic category and calculating the evocation capacities. As a result greater 'consistency' between (expressions of) evocation capacities and 'matching' is expected.

Given a prototype E_1 ($\ldots$ At_i $\ldots$) and the patient datum E_1' ($\ldots$ At_i' $\ldots$), attempts were made to calculate a degree of 'conformity' between the attributes At_i and At_i' between the values 0 and 1; where 0 means complete dissimilarity and 1 that they are identical. It is noted that this degree of semantic conformity may only be calculated for two expressions of the same entity, two parts being semantically comparable on condition that they have the same language field.

The degree t is based on the semantic category tree and is calculated empirically as follows:

$t = 1$ IF $At_i = At_i'$

In other words the At_i' values of the attribute are equal or like:
$At_i' = $ DEPENDANT OF At_i

$$t = 1 - \frac{1}{(n + 1)^2)} \text{ IF } At_i = \text{DEPENDANT-OF}$$

$$t = 1 - \frac{1}{n + 1} \text{ In the other cases}$$

where n refers to the founder or common predecessor at At_i and At'_i.

Table 3.1 gives values of t obtained from data of the semantic category described above. It will be observed that the table is not symmetrical just like the 'matching' operation which it represents. Table 3.1 values of t for 'Change in appetite'.

If the symptom is described by several attributes the expert applies a weighting for each one during development of the system to express its evoking power.

Once t is evaluated the evocation force is calculated from the evoking capacity e (weighted between 0 and 1), allocated to the prototype by the expert, and t. The evocation force is given by:

$$= Max(t + e - 1, 0) \qquad 0 \leqslant \alpha \leqslant 1$$

similarly, the rejection force B is calculated from t' and r, the rejection

Table 3.1 Values of 't' for the attribute 'change of appetite'

$\langle At_i \rangle$ \ $\langle At'_i \rangle$	I	II	III	IV	V	VI	VII
I = INCREASED	1	1	1	0	0	0	0
II = MARKEDLY INCREASED	0.75	1	0.5	0	0	0	0
III = SLIGHTLY INCREASED	0.75	0.5	1	0	0	0	0
IV = NORMAL	0	0	0	1	0	0	0
V = DECREASED	0	0	0	0	1	1	1
VI = MARKEDLY DECREASED	0	0	0	0	0.75	1	0.5
VII = SLIGHTLY DECREASED	0	0	0	0	0.75	0.5	1

Value for:

n

0

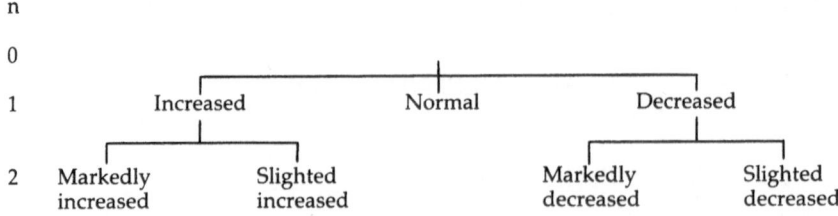

force (weighted between 0 and 1) assigned by the expert; t' for calculation of B being the homologue of t.

$$B = Min(t' + 1 - r, 1) \qquad 0 \leqslant \beta \leqslant 1$$

The simultaneous occurrence of these two results leads, when there is no disagreement (i.e. when $\alpha < \beta$) between any symptom with evocation and rejection power in the various contexts, to a space $[\alpha, \beta]$ within whose limits choice of diagnostic direction may be made.

Example:

The expert provides this knowledge:
APPETITE (Greatly reduced) EVOKES (0.6) CTX CHANGE IN GENERAL STATE
APPETITE (Reduced) REJECTS (0.1) CTX CHANGE IN GENERAL STATE

(note that the calculation of β reduces the second assertion to: absence of reduced appetite rejects with a force 0.1 a context of change in general state)

The patient presents the following symptom:
APPETITE (Reduced)

The gap $[\alpha, \beta]$ allows calculation of the evocation and rejection of the symptom for a change in context of the general state as follows:

$$\alpha = Max(t + e - 1, 0) = Max(0.75 + 0.6 - 1, 0) = 0.35$$
$$\beta = Min(t' - r + 1, 1) = Min(1 + 1 - 0.1, 1) = 1$$
$$\text{where the interval is } (0.35; 1)$$

From the size of this space it can be said that APPETITE (Reduced) leaves fairly serious uncertainty over direction of 'change in general condition context', even though the lower limit is raised to 0.35, which implies that there are some elements which support this orientation.

The fact that the upper limit remains at 1 means that there is nothing to prove that one is not faced with a pathology which takes place in a change in general state context.

The intervals $[\alpha_i^j, \beta_i^j]$ are calculated for each entity E_i and each context j. The interval a_j, b_j is constructed to typify the evocation and the rejection of a given context, j:

$$(a_j = \underset{i}{Max} \; \alpha_i^j \qquad b_j = \underset{i}{min} \; \beta_i^j)$$

The choice of context then reduces to the one with an interval a_j; b_j it will depend upon the context j and meet the following criterion:

$$\text{Max}_j = \frac{a_j + b_j}{2}$$

In the case where several intervals might have the same mean the one which has the highest lower limits is chosen. If there is disagreement as, for instance, where $\alpha > \beta$ then the interval $(0, \beta)$ is selected; that is, only the rejection force is taken into account and the evocation force is disregarded.

The following results were obtained from the application to the diagnosis of jaundice, which have been classified into nine contexts:

1. That of distress which amalgamates diagnoses or clinical forms into emergency schedules.
2. The painful context dominated by the symptom of pain.
3. The congenital anaemia context.
4. The chronic anaemia context.
5. The infectious context.
6. The encephalopathy context.
7. The change in general state context.
8. The iatrogenic context.
9. The cholestasis context.

Example One

A boy aged 14 years presented with the following symptoms at consultation:

NORMAL TEMPERATURE AND SUBICTERIC FOR 2 MONTHS
URINE: NORMAL COLOUR
STOOL: NORMAL COLOUR
PALPABLE SPLEEN; NORMAL LIVER, SMOOTH, PAINLESS

Evocation results

Distress context	0.00	0.19
Painful context	0.00	0.40
Congenital anaemia context	0.40	0.60
Chronic amaemia context	0.39	0.39
Infectious context	0.09	0.30
Encephalopathy context	0.00	0.19
Change in general state context	0.09	0.10

Iatrogenic context	0.00	0.50
Cholestasis context	0.00	0.50

In this case, the two contexts chosen are:

1. Congenital anaemia context
2. Chronic anaemia context

Example Two

At consultation a woman aged 39 years presented with
RECENT FRANK JAUNDICE ACCOMPANIED BY MODERATE
   PRURITIS
NO PAIN
ON ORAL CONTRACEPTIVES AND ALDOMET

Evocation results

Distress context	0.00	0.00
Painful context	0.29	0.40
Congenital anaemia context	0.09	0.40
Chronic amaemia context	0.09	0.70
Infectious context	0.09	0.70
Encephalopathy context	0.20	0.50
Change in general state context	0.09	0.70
Iatrogenic context	0.50	1.00
Cholestasis context	0.50	0.50

Here, the two contexts chosen are (in the order):

1. Iatrogenic context
2. Cholestasis context

Example Three

A patient aged 40 years presented with the following symptoms at consultation:

PALLOR
SUBICTERIC FOR 1 MONTH
ALCOHOLISM
NORMAL TEMPERATURE
NO PAIN

Evocation results

Distress context	0.00	0.19
Painful context	0.00	0.39
Congenital anaemia context	0.30	0.30
Chronic anaemia context	0.50	1.00
Infectious context	0.09	0.30
Encephalopathy context	0.30	0.80
Change in general state context	0.19	1.00
Iatrogenic context	0.00	0.50
Cholestasis context	0.34	0.50

In this case the applicable choice of context is first chronic anaemia and in second place, change in general state.

3.5.4   Control: agenda, meta-knowledge and meta-rules

There are two distinct components of the control system: first, production of the agenda, its development, evolution and scrutiny; the second component is connected with triggering of forward or reverse chaining rules, the use of conflict resolution rules and to the implicit control linked to the expression of the knowledge rules premises.

The agenda

Control of SPHINX is based mainly on the list of tasks to be performed during the consultation. At the start of the consultation the agenda is provided with a single task, to carry out the evocation; when this has been achieved those tasks which are pertinent to the evoked contexts are added to the agenda in the order in which they appear in the context definition, the same order in which SPHINX will try to carry them out (FIFO). The expert, therefore, when he lists the elements of a context such as diagnoses and therapies, arranges the tasks according to a context-linked criterion; for example, in a cold cholestasis context, he might enumerate the possible diagnoses in terms of their frequency in this particular clinical picture, whereas in a distress context, lines of research might be indicated by assessment of the severity and urgency of the process. Performance of any task included in the agenda may lead to changes in (its) content through triggering of rules with actions such as:

1. TO THINK OF: This permits a goal or a list of goals to be added to the task list in the agenda without interrupting the task in

progress. The objective is added at the end and will therefore be considered last.

2. TO LOOK FOR: Causes interruption of pursuit of the objective in progress and suggests another task to the System.
3. TO IGNORE: Allows quite different diagnosis to be put into practice by deleting the elements in the goals list.
4. TO ASK FOR: Enables one test or several complementary tests to be requested at any given time; without changing the agenda contents.

SPHINX will perform all the tasks and try to achieve all the goals on the agenda. Its main role is to make the control accessible and explicit; in particular, it allows display of the goals proposed by the system, provision of the goals in check: an outline, as it were, of the SPHINX reasoning which leads to development of a module which explains the system behaviour; as, for example, in CENTAUR.

The meta knowledge

It concerns the use of all the knowledge available to the system. A meta-knowledge component can be recognized in the definition of contexts and in the use of evocation rules and test rules each triggered in forward chaining, or in the use of conflict resolution rules. The very expression rules entails some implicit control and this aspect will be considered. Gascuel (1981) distinguishes two forms of meta-rules: those provided by the user to replace some rules in a context where they would be applicable; and, the strategic meta-rules which do not change the meaning of the rules when specifying their application context, but are rapid ways of letting the user avoid unnecessary schedules. While this binary division seems to simplify the problem and is endorsed, it is emphasized that the separation of the meta-knowledge rules and the knowledge rules recommended by Davis (1980b) has not been researched, but the control entry integrated in the interpreter is restricted as much as possible so that the expert may change the system strategy by modification of the rules and contexts. The various elements of the meta-knowledge and their use in the system will now be discussed.

The meta-rules The meta-rules allow the system strategy to be modified and in both SPHINX and EMYCIN are capable of operating on other rules, particularly on the list of rules which lead to attainment of a sub-goal, directing this list and deleting rules from it.

Example: Conflict resolution rules such as:

Rule 1: IF EVALUATION (Rule, TRUE) THEN TO TRIGGER (Rule)

Rule 2: IF EVALUATION (Rule FALSE) THEN DISCARD (Rule)

Rule 3: IF LIST (empty) THEN DEMONSTRATION (goal, CHECK) AND TO CHANGE (goal)

Rule 4: IF LIST (not empty) THEN TO CONTROL AND DEMONSTRATION (goal, TO INITIATE)

Use of these four rules every time a rule is selected to reach a goal operates a mechanism identical to the prevision of EMYCIN; so before considering a rule which is applicable, the user satisfies himself that none of the premise clauses is already known and at variance with the data base, in which case it will be ELIMINATED (rule 2).

Example:

	Knowledge base:	Facts base:
C_1	$A_\wedge B_\wedge C \rightarrow D$	A
C_2	$A_\wedge E_\wedge F \rightarrow D$	$\rceil E$
C_3	$G_\wedge H_\wedge F \rightarrow D$	B
C_4	$B_\wedge K_\wedge E \rightarrow D$	
C_5	$L_\wedge M_\wedge N \rightarrow K$	

Rule 2 eliminates C_2 and C_4 from the list of applicable rules to achieve D given the above facts base.

In certain cases the use of rule 2 saves looking for a symptom or requesting a test. In the preceding example it is the entity K which is used solely by the knowledge rule C_4; and because of E amongst the data, C_4 is eliminated from the list of possible rules and the system will not be interested in K, which results in suppression of questions which would not be relevant to the patient's condition. This rule therefore allows elimination of irrelevant sub-goals and avoids questions on entities L, M and N.

Rule 1 sees that there are insufficient elements in the data base to achieve the desired goal on account of one rule. All the SPHINX rules allow a conclusion to be reached with certainty (CF = 1); as soon as a rule permits the goal to be reached it is immediately applied and the other pertinent rules are not tested. This procedure of working through sufficient terms for goal attainment means that one eliminates a number of questions, and searches for entities which lead to the same conclusion as a consultation where only the relevant questions are asked. This way of triggering rules still poses a problem in some cases which is demonstrated in the following example:

Knowledge base	Data base
(C_1) $A_\wedge B_\wedge C \rightarrow D$	A
(C_2) $A_\wedge E_\wedge F \rightarrow D_\wedge G$	B
	C

According to meta-rule 1, the knowledge rule C_1 may be triggered through the data base without asking the user any questions. As a result, D is added to the data base and the user does not attempt to trigger C_2. It can be seen that if G appears on the agenda, C_2 is tested to achieve G, but only if G is listed. It is in fact rare to affirm two different diagnoses at the same time from a single rule; this did not occur in the jaundice case. On the contrary it often happens that the fact of affirming a diagnosis allows a differential diagnosis to be made within the same rule by discarding others through the action TO IGNORE.

This case has not presented a problem since the diagnoses appearing in the action TO IGNORE have a sufficiently related symptomatology to the diagnosis to confirm that they happen to be in the same context. It is therefore while seeking to carry out the agenda tasks that the differential diagnosis rules may be considered; thus, in the example above, if G signifies TO IGNORE VIRAL HEPATITIS B, it may be thought that D is a disease with a symptomatology akin to viral hepatitis B, so after demonstration of D, VIRAL HEPATITIS B is added to the agenda. This form of hepatitis is listed in rule C_2.

After application of meta-rules 1 and 2, if the list of possible rules is not empty, meta-rule 4 is used to select a rule from several others. This choice is made according to which entities occur in the premises and to the value assigned to their attribute. The attribute coding follows the order:

	Interrogation sign	Clinical examination sign	Paraclinical result	Diagnosis
Level:	1	2	3	4

The first rule to test is chosen according to its (position) level (disregarding those entities which may already appear in the data base). For the rule:

$A_\wedge B_\wedge C \rightarrow D$
(then level (Rule) = level $(A_\wedge B_\wedge C)$ = Max (level A), level (B), level (C)).

The choice rests with the rule having the lowest level; in the case where several rules present in the same level it is classified by the minimum number of entities determining the level of each rule.

Other components of meta-knowledge

1. Antecedent rules
Both evocation rules and rules for interpreting complementary tests are triggered in forward chaining and refer to actions affecting the agenda.

> Examples:
> (1) IF: CHILD
>   MILD JAUNDICE
>   PALLOR
> THEN:
>   TO EVOKE: CONGENITAL ANAEMIA CONTEXT
>   IF: HAEMOGLOBIN REDUCED
>   NORMOCHROMIA
>   RETICULOCYTES RAISED
> THEN:
>   FN: REGENERATIVE NORMOCHROMIC
>   ANAEMIA
>   TO THINK OF: HAEMOGLOBINOPATHY
>   AUTO-IMMUNE ANAEMIA

It is evident that these elements of pure knowledge are intimately linked to the meta-knowledge in the same rules, as such a representation seems more natural to the expert. These elements of meta-knowledge are in fact intricately involved with the knowledge and it would have been quite unnatural to want to separate them; in addition, it would lead to an unjustifiable increase in the number of rules and a slow-down due to their consultation.

2. Differential diagnosis rules

Example:

> Rule 117: IF: SUBICTERIC
>   ENLARGED SPLEEN
>   FREE BILIRUBIN PREDOMINANT(LY)
>   FN: IRON-DEFICIENT ANAEMIA
>   BLOOD IRON INCREASED
>   ELECTROPHORESIS: THALASSAEMIC
>   HAEMOGLOBIN
>   THEN: HAEMOGLOBINOPATHY: THALASSAEMIA
>   TO THINK OF: LITHIASIS
>   CIRRHOSIS
>   TO IGNORE: MINKOWSKI-CHAUFFARD
>   ENZYMATIC DEFICIENCY

Like the previous rules, these include meta-knowledge components which allow for change in the agenda, especially to cut down the task list. They are activated in reverse chaining with regard to the goals which are directly evident in their 'effect' parts; or, for diagnostic entities controlled by the Verb TO IGNORE (rule 117 will be taken into consideration if the proposed task is either HAEMOGLOBINOPATHY, THALASSAEMIA, MINKOWSKI-CHAUFFARD or ENZYMATIC DEFICIENCY). If the diagnostic goals directed by the verb TO IGNORE do not appear on the agenda they are added to the list and confined like goals in check.

3. Elements of implicit control
Part of the knowledge used in the control is provided implicitly by the wording of the rules. In fact, the order in which the literals occur in the rule fix the order in which they will be asked for by the user. The expert must therefore take account of this implicit control element when representing his knowledge. For example, where clinical and paraclinical data are present in a rule it is advisable to list all the clinical entities as principal components of the condition part, in the order, according to their sensitivity and specificity, in which they would be requested by the user for as coherent a dialogue as possible. Attention has been drawn in the previous chapter to the difficulties of safeguarding a 'conversation logic' in the behaviour of a system of production rules triggered in reverse chaining. In fact, the development of questions is consistent with the course of the AND/OR tree which corresponds to the rules, but the backtracking entailed by checks in the pursuit of sub-aims sometimes leads to questions on clinical symptoms after looking for paraclinical signs. This works against the advantage offered by representation of the knowledge in the form of modular and independent production rules. The control may be modified in certain cases; for example, in EMYCIN use of the Verb TO ASK FOR plays essentially the same role as ASK FIRST or INITIAL DATA. Similarly, the expert may insert entities into the evocation rules whose attributes are not fixed; that is, entities which do not strictly speaking introduce conditions, but whose appearance in the rule premise results in the initial question to the user at the start of the consultation. Such entities play the same role as defined parameters like INITIAL DATA in EMYCIN.

Example:
In the following evocation rule the entities AGE and SEX appear solely because the user was asked and have no effect on the triggering of the rule:

    IF: AGE
            SEX

URGENT ADMISSION
STATE OF SHOCK
THEN:
TO EVOKE: CTXT DISTRESS

Similarly, part of the control of the questions put to the user is assumed by MEDIUM. This is true in several situations:

1. One entity is linked to others for the evaluation of its attributes.

Example: the number of Red Cells depends on age and sex. In this case MEDIUM takes the initiative to ask questions on all the entities concerned.

2. One entity forming part of a complementary examination: in this case MEDIUM asks all the entities concerned in the examination itself whether an EXPERT would be interested *a priori* in just one of them in the rule in process.

The possibilities offered by SPHINX allow better organization of questions and a dialogue which is both more consistent and more relevant.

3.6   DISCUSSION

SPHINX has been provided with the capability of referring to and using two types of knowledge: an approximate knowledge and a certain knowledge. The savoir faire and experience which allows total appreciation of a clinical situation without well-defined objective criteria is interpreted by heuristics, making use of large amounts of data which by their very nature and mode of acquisition have an indirect effect on the choice of formalism used to express them. This method of representing an heuristic knowledge to achieve evocation, like an approximate knowledge allowing formulation of the hypotheses which limit the research field, approximates to the techniques used in PIP. Certain knowledge is represented by non-weighted production rules even though most of the currently operational systems use rules endued with credibility factors to draw their conclusions. It is worth noting that, like SPHINX, SACON does not use ponderation factors for its rules. Van Melle (1980) emphasizes that the CFs of MYCIN are such that small variations of the CF of a rule do not give result in a great difference in the final result. The system remains consistent if the CF is expressed on a scale of from four to six certainty values (0.0, 0.2, 0.4, 0.6, 0.8, 1.0, for example). These CFs may be thought of as simplifying elements which enable the knowledge to be expressed in propositional form in the rules. Use of a logic dependent on the domain in SPHINX produces more powerful language which enables CF to be dispensed with in the applications envisaged. Non-weighted rules bring about a much greater modularity in the knowledge representation, because of the absence of reinforcement of one rule by another. This makes it possible for a knowledge base to be developed by several experts, difficult to devise in a MYCIN-type system where the interactions of one rule on another may assume great significance and where, as a result, one expert alone may modify the system with full knowledge of the facts. However, as emphasized earlier as soon as a goal is reached through triggering of a rule the system ignores the other rules which lead to this same goal and, the actions which may be associated with them. This problem is linked to the search for enough conditions to reach a goal. Although in practice no difficulty has been encountered with this strategy, a way of improving it will be sought to avoid the need to enact hand-written rules for the knowledge. Their unique and straightforward syntax and total independence seems to come close to our ways of thinking which facilitates the task of the experts particularly in production of the knowledge base.

One further point connected with the formalism and the representation of the production rules merits attention; it concerns the context elements implicit in the rules of such systems as MYCIN, some of which may be written in the following way:

IF $A_\wedge B_\wedge D$ THEN C_1
IF $A_\wedge B_\wedge E$ THEN C_2
IF $A_\wedge B_\wedge F$ THEN C_3

A and B may be considered in this case as context elements for determining the value of D, E or F. For example, to appreciate the number of red cells (RC) age and sex should be considered; in a system like MYCIN inclusion of these two entities would be repeated in the rules as:

R_1 IF (RC $\geqslant$ 4.5) AND (RC $\leqslant$ 6) AND (AGE $\geqslant$ 16) AND (SEX MALE) ... THEN ...
R_2 IF (RC $\geqslant$ 4) AND (RC $\leqslant$ 5.5) AND (AGE $\geqslant$ 16) AND (SEX FEMALE) ... THEN ...
R_3 IF (RC $>$ 6) AND (AGE $\geqslant$ 16) AND (SEX MALE) ... THEN ...

MEDIUM uses a knowledge which allows EXPERT to work solely in symbols, which has the advantage of defining the concepts of normal, increased or reduced RC, bearing in mind relevant entities such as age and sex. Thus, part of the valuation of symptoms context is undertaken by MEDIUM, which allows for more synthetic and concise writing of the production rules, not dealing with this problem of context; this makes them easier to read and understand so approaching the representation of VM (Fagan *et al.*, 1979). As a result, the rules R_1 and R_2 referred to above, merged for SPHINX, if they have the same conclusion, into a single rule:

IF RC Normal … THEN …

Likewise, rule R_3 would be in the form:

IF RC Increased … THEN …

This integration of contextual elements, allowing some patient's symptoms to be appreciated, seems more flexible than that used particularly in CENTAUR, where the rules are combined in the contexts and activated provided these are verified. The structuring of the rules found in the CENTAUR solution for clarifying the context runs counter to the desired modularity, introduces very great developmental difficulties and seems to have rather limited application, like that of PUFF-CENTAUR, in order that the contexts may be defined by prototypes.

Since EXPERT communicates with MEDIUM making SPHINX an interactive system it was natural to provide for data-directed control operated in forward chaining. This need has been foreseen through the evocation and examination rules which allow the system to behave strictly with regard to patient data, without becoming stereotyped. The feasibility of working in reverse chaining avoids considering numerous rules unconnected with the patient's state and requires fewer symptoms and examinations to be pursued. This need for control seems close enough to that of medical experts. The conflict resolution rules allow the control to be refined and to focus the deductive mechanism, as in EMYCIN or TEIRESIAS. As a result, the forecast mechanism enables the user to anticipate without trying the rules, some of whose premise components are false, and avoids asking pointless questions.

Another aspect of the interactive system concerns the detection of inconsistent or contradictory data. SPHINX is capable of detecting various types of inconsistencies. A sign may be inherently at variance or with respect to the program knowledge (incompatibility with a physiological knowledge for instance). A number of red cells, equal to 100 000 per ml, represents the first type of inconsistency. It is detected on entry and can be corrected by asking the user the question again. The second type of contradiction derives from a discrepancy between the various entities in the data and knowledge base. For example, the conjugated bilirubin concentration is greatly raised without clinical jaundice. In this case the order of appearance of the signs in the data base has a significant effect on the behaviour of the system; in fact, the system recalls the entity that introduces the inconsistency, which is the last one supplied to the system. This way of coping with contradictions does not simplify the problem much and is not entirely satisfactory. It would be advantageous to be able to delete any entity involved in the contradiction (which might eventually become a conclusion deduced by the system) and to withdraw from the data base all conclusions which might derive from this entity. This touches on a taxing problem, to which Gallaire has drawn attention, regarding deductive data bases, where division between integrity rules, which ensure consistency, and rules of deduction, which allow inference from data, are not always clear (Kowalski, 1977).

Minsky has generally reviewed logical theories which, contrary to natural language, obey the extension property characteristic of monotony; that is if a set of rules S is such that $S \rightarrow p$ and $S \subseteq S'$ then $S' \rightarrow p$. As a result, use of exception rules or rules of conjuncture (McCarthy, 1982) may be especially relevant in medicine and may be considered as a refinement to the proposed model. This system would use a set of rules, leading to conclusions open to modification by rules representing the special cases and the exceptions. This fascinating problem must become the subject of an in-depth study for the future version of SPHINX.

Finally, a brief return to the explanation capabilities of Artificial Intelligence methods and systems like SPHINX. If this asset has been frequently promoted it is above all to stress the ability of these systems to provide the rules on which their conclusions rest. In our opinion, it is essential to go further and provide these systems with truly explanatory rules since the production rules written for decision-making may not be appropriate. For example, a rule may express a very detailed knowledge of several entities which conceals (or implies) a basic physiological principle or underlying physiopathology which is needed to explain and to return to through explanation rules. The formalism of production rules readily permits this. To write: a because b leads to the rule IF b THEN a. Continuation of this work in computer-assisted development in medicine should be set in this perspective.

4
Examples of applications

4.1 APPLICATION TO THE DIAGNOSTIC AID FOR JAUNDICE

4.1.1 Contexts

Nine contexts have been defined for this application; nine general 'clinical frameworks' for promoting diagnostic hypotheses that Pople (1982) calls intermediary pathological specifications which characterize and manipulate the patient's symptomatology. Each context bears the name of the symptom, the syndrome or the condition which describes the clinical state of the patient as follows:

1. painful context
2. distress context
3. congenital anaemia context
4. chronic anaemia context
5. infectious context
6. encephalopathy context
7. change of general state context
8. iatrogenic context
9. cholestatis context.

The painful context is characterized mainly by jaundice accompanied by a pain, in which context the following diagnostic hypotheses are recognized: lithiasis, angiocholitis, cancer of the pancreas, cancer of the liver, pancreatitis, cardiac liver, hepatic abscess, hydatid cyst, poisoning.

The distress context is evoked first of all if there is jaundice together with an emergency or serious symptom such as coma, any consciousness disorder, intestinal haemmorhage, or haemoglobinuria; the diagnostic hypotheses are then: septicaemia, transfusion accidents, malaria, haemoglobinopathy, enzyme deficiency, immuno-allergic anaemia, poisoning.

One diagnosis may appear in several contexts; thus malaria will be found again in the context of chronic anaemia. The appearance of the same disease in several contexts corresponds to the number of its clinical forms: in the distress context malaria is a pernicious attack, whereas in the chronic anaemia context it is a commonplace condition. When a child with the congenital anaemia context presents with pallor, asthenia or a large spleen, one of three etiologies may be considered: haemoglobinopathy, Minkowski-Chauffard's Syndrome or an enzyme deficiency such as Griggler-Najjar disease, Gilbert disease, favism or pyruvate kinase deficiency.

Symptoms of anaemia considered in the chronic anaemia context include the following diagnoses: cirrhosis, Addison Biermer anaemia, auto-immune anaemia, malignant haemopathy, malaria, mechanical anaemia and poisoning.

Jaundice associated with a temperature above 38° would favour an infectious context including: cholangitis, septicaemia, hepatitis, cancer of the liver, malaria, liver abscess and hydatid cyst.

Encephalopathy context is characterized by mood disorders, asterixis, and consciousness disorders comprising diagnoses of cirrhosis, cancer of the liver, hepatitis, poisoning and acute steatosis of pregnancy.

Definition of the general change of state context rests mainly on anorexia, weight loss and asthenia with classified diagnoses of cancer of the liver, cancer of the pancreas, cirrhosis, cancer of the gall bladder, cancer of the bile ducts, cancer of the ampulla of Vater, cardiac liver and benign tumour of the common bile duct.

The iatrogenic context implies involvement of medical dosage or existence of mechanical causes such as valve carriers. The following diagnoses are classified in this context: hepatitis, medical cholestasis and mechanical anaemia. The first two diagnoses are involved in their medical forms.

The cholestasis context is considered regarding dark urine, discoloured stools and pruritis, and comprises the following diagnoses: hepatitis, cancer of the liver, cancer of the pancreas, cirrhosis, lithiasis, pancreatitis, cancer of the gall bladder, cancer of the ampulla of Vater and benign tumour of the common bile duct.

The diagnoses in each context are given in an order which takes account of the frequency of the disease and/or its gravity.

4.1.2 The rules

In its application to the diagnosis of jaundice the system uses about four hundred rules; half of these comprise interpretation of test rules while the other half allow requests for complementary tests and affirmation of diagnoses; more than fifteen rules enable the evocations to be triggered. An example of each type of rule will follow.

Evocation rule:

IF   PATIENT SEEN AS EMERGENCY
        EMERGENCY CASE
        INTESTINAL HAEMORRHAGE
THEN TO EVOKE ENCEPHALOPATHY CONTEXT

Diagnostic decision rule:

IF   SUBICTERUS
        UNCONJUGATED BILIRUBIN MAINLY
        IRON-DEFICIENT
        INCREASED BLOOD IRON
        HAEMOGLOBIN ELECTROPHORESIS:
                        THALASSAEMIA
THEN THALASSAEMIC HAEMOGLOBINOPATHY
        TO THINK OF: LITHIASIS
                        CIRRHOSIS
        TO IGNORE: MINKOWSKI-CHAUFFARD
                        ENZYME DEFICIENCY

Test interpretation rule:

IF   HAEMOGLOBIN: ANAEMIA
        HYPOCHROMIA
        MICROCYTOSIS
THEN   IRON DEFICIENCY
        TO IGNORE: PERNICIOUS ANAEMIA

Close on 250 entities have been defined and used for this application.

4.1.3   Example of a consultation

The shortest consultation time is 12 minutes on a MITRA 225 working in shared time.

The following development of a SPHINX consultation concerns a patient record used in the validation of the jaundice diagnostic aid (application). Text denoted by M: are from the machine; text in lower case is provided by the user (U:) either spontaneously or in reply to a question from the system; and texts in italic script are comments on the consultation or its development.

SPHINX:
    M: ON WHICH APPLICATION DO YOU WANT TO WORK?
    U: Man of 38 years
    U: Severe asthenia for 3 months
    U: Anorexia for 3 months
    U: Weight loss
    M: HOW SIGNIFICANT (IN KG)?
    U: 20
    U: Profuse and frequent vomiting for 4 days
    M: WAS IT PROMPTED BY CERTAIN CIRCUMSTANCES?
    U: No
    U: No pain
    U: Normal temperature
    U: Frank jaundice for 8 days
    U: Dark urine for 8 days
    M: WHAT IS THE MEAN DAILY VOLUME OF URINE?
    U: Normal
    U: No pruritis
    U: Stop

'Stop' indicates that the user has no more spontaneous information for the machine. While allowing freedom of expression of the complaint, the system sometimes asked questions to specify attributes of certain entities, for example, the significance of the weight loss. Using these data SPHINX continues its attempts to carry out its assignment.

    M: IS THE PATIENT'S CONTEXT KNOWN?
    U: Yes
    M: IS A CONSULTATION INVOLVED?
    U: Yes

SPHINX does not achieve the evocation and completes it through some questions designed to provide sufficient data to trigger an evocation rule.

    M: ARE CONSCIOUSNESS DISORDERS DETECTED?
    U: No

At this stage SPHINX triggers an evocation rule, a heuristic procedure: the system agenda from now on contains the goals: hepatitis, cancer of the liver, cancer of the pancreas, cirrhosis, lithiasis, pancreatitis, cancer of the bladder, cancer of the bile ducts, cancer of the ampulla of Vater, benign tumour of the common bile duct and cardiac liver.

M: HAS THE LIVER BEEN EXAMINED?
U: Yes
M: HOW IS IT ON PALPITATION?
U: Enlarged
M: HOW DOES IT APPEAR?
U: Smooth
M: IS IT PAINFUL?
U: No
M: WAS THE GALL-BLADDER EXAMINED?
U: Yes
M: IS THE BLADDER ENLARGED?
U: No
M: IS THERE A MURPHY'S SIGN?
U: No
U: Spleen not palpable

At this stage in the consultation, the user may provide data either in response to the system or spontaneously, as in the case of the information concerning the spleen.

M: HAS THE BILIRUBIN BEEN MEASURED?
U: Yes
M: WHAT IS THE UNCONJUGATED BILIRUBIN CONCENTRA-
   TION (MICROMOL/L)?
U: 34
M: WHAT IS THE CONJUGATED BILIRUBIN CONCENTRA-
   TION (MICROMOL/L)?
U: 85
M: WHAT IS THE TOTAL BILIRUBIN CONCENTRATION
   (MICROMOL/L)?
U: 119
M: HAVE THE TRANSAMINASES BEEN MEASURED?
U: Yes
M: WHAT IS THE SGOT (IU/L)?
U: 59
M: WHAT IS THE SGPT (IU/L)?
U: 57
U: ?
M: PRESENT CONDITION
M: SGPT CONCENTRATION: RAISED
M: O.K.?
U: Yes

The reply '?' from the user results in visual display of the system interpretation of the last entity considered, which is followed by the question O.K.? If the reply is 'no' the entity in question is withdrawn, otherwise the consultation continues:

M: IS THERE A PREVIOUS HISTORY OF HEPATITIS?
U: Yes
M: HOW LONG AGO?
U: 3 months
M: WHAT IS THE TYPE OF DEVELOPMENT OF THE HEPATITIS?
U: Acute
M: WHAT IS THE AETIOLOGY OF THE HEPATITIS?
U: B
U: No previous history of diabetes
U: No alcoholism
U: No smoking

Here the machine asks a question of great significance to the final diagnosis, as will be seen later on. Also, the user, although not requested by the machine, has completed the information of the previous history regarding diabetes, alcohol and smoking.

M: HAS AUSTRALIA ANTIGEN BEEN LOOKED FOR?
U: Yes
M: PRESENT OR ABSENT
U: Present
M: HAS THE GALL-BLADDER BEEN SCANNED?
U: No
U: No liver scan
M: ARE THE ALPHA-2-GLOBULINS KNOWN?
U: Yes
M: ALPHA-2-GLOBULINS (%)?
U: Alpha-1   24.3
U: Beta   5.5
U: Gamma   46.1
U: Albumin 38

The machine starts to ask for the electrophoresis results. The user gives it all the results without waiting to be asked for them. Were this not the case the system, which is informed of the electrophoresis test, would have carried on with the relevant questions.

M: HAS THE PROTHROMBIN (CONCENTRATION) BEEN MEASURED?
U: Yes

M: WHAT IS THE PT TIME?
U: 50
M: IS THERE ANY EVIDENCE OF BILIARY COLIC?
U: No
M: HAS THE ALPHA-FOETO-PROTEIN BEEN MEASURED?
U: No
M: IS ASCITES PRESENT?
U: Yes, laminal ascites
M: TO CARRY OUT: FIBROSCOPY
                  PBH
U: No fibroscopy
M: SUSPECTED HEPATITIS
M: SUSPECTED CIRRHOSIS
M: SUSPECTED CANCER OF THE LIVER
M: POST-HEPATIC CIRRHOSIS

The consultation comes to an end with visual display of the system diagnosis of POST-HEPATIC CIRRHOSIS worked out after having suspected hepatitis, cirrhosis and cancer of the liver.

4.1.4   Initial validation results

These are set out in Bruchet's thesis (1983). This preliminary study was carried out on fifty medical case histories taken at random from Professor Salducci's gastro-enterology department at the Nord Hospital at Marseille. All the records were complete and with verified diagnoses.

In each case SPHINX was provided with the functional and general recall signs from the admission card. During the consultation, replies were produced in accordance with the content of the medical record. This procedure provided the results presented in Table 4.1, which should be considered as a preliminary study since the sample came from only one hospital department. This has prevented testing the system knowledge on cases of jaundice originating from a haematological problem. Moreover, the trial records used to improve part of the system knowledge were obtained from the same department as those used in the preliminary study. This ensures that the particular skills of this gastro-enterology department have directed the writing of the knowledge rules, according to the prescribed practices and the development of the collection of routine complementary tests carried out in the department. It would be worthwhile evaluating the results of the current knowledge from records from other departments or from local general practitioners.

In many cases the diagnoses affirmed by the system were more accurate than Table 4.1 indicates; for example, of the eight cases of viral

Table 4.1 Preliminary results of validation of the diagnosis of the cause of jaundice

Expert's diagnosis	Number of cases	SPHINX diagnosis	Cases not diagnosed by SPHINX
Viral hepatitis	8	8	—
Drug induced hepatitis	2	1	1
Alcoholic hepatitis	2	2	—
Chronic hepatitis	2	1	1
Alcoholic cirrhosis	4	4	—
Cirrhosis (other causes)	3	3	—
Decompensated cirrhosis	2	2	—
Cholangitis	4	4	—
Liver cancer	3	3	—
Cancer of pancreas	4	4	—
Carcinoma of bile duct	2	2	—
Gall stones	5	5	—
Carcinoma of ampalla of vater	1	1	—
Chronic pancreatitis	4	3	1
Others	4	3	1

hepatitis, the system recognized four viral hepatitis B, three viral hepatitis A and one which could not be classified because the serology was not available. The heading 'others' combines a hydatid cyst, an amoebic abscess and two cardiac livers, one of which was not discovered by the machine.

It happens that the system may not reach a conclusion in which case it does not propose any diagnosis: in no case has an erroneous diagnosis been obtained. This is an important characteristic which helps to improve the program knowledge and its behaviour by encouraging inclusion of supplementary rules. In this respect, it differs from other approaches, such as the probabilist model, which allow a few false conclusions as a necessary consequence of the model (Szolovits and Long, 1982).

This initial evaluation is placed on a par with the first version of the system which constitutes a feasibility study. A more rigorous evaluation of its performance and acceptability by the users should follow.

4.2 APPLICATION TO THERAPEUTIC AID IN THE TREATMENT OF DIABETES

If the results of an enquiry carried out on five hundred general practitioners from the Provence-Alpes-Cote d'Azur regions and Corsica are to be believed, then 70% of the doctors who replied were fully aware of the problems that they face in diabetic therapy; and 75% declared interest in the experimental use of an information system in this domain.

Diabetes is nevertheless a commonplace disorder against which our entire therapeutic arsenal comprises three types of drug: insulin, the biguanides and the sulphamides; and calorie and glucide-controlled diet. The control methods are simple since they are limited usually to blood glucose and acetests. However, to treat a diabetic is by no means straightforward; it demands a great deal of data and the experienced doctor plays a central role.

In France between one million and one million and a half patients suffer from diabetes, of whom about 12% are insulin-dependent which highlights the magnitude of the problem this disease presents to the Health Service, and the benefit that an operational decision-aid system in this domain would offer.

4.2.1   The contexts

The three following contexts were defined for this application:

1. Insulin
2. Biguanide
3. Sulphamide

The choice of context depends on whether the patient is already being treated with insulin, biguanides or sulphamides but also, mainly on the age of the patient, the degree of obesity or the lack of equilibration.

For each context, the system can be directed to consider these therapeutic goals: to apply appropriate resuscitation, to administer an initial treatment (insulin, biguanide or sulphamide), to advocate a diet or withdraw therapy, to advise continuation of the previous treatment or to propose a change of treatment and dose.

The value of the contexts is less evident here where the problem posed is much more limited than in the case of jaundice. In fact, only about ten entities are needed to make a decision in the most difficult cases and, save in rare exceptions, all these entities concern decision-making no matter what the case. However, these contexts set a limit on the number of rules required.

4.2.2   The rules

The system uses about three hundred rules of which about fifty are triggered in forward chaining.

Examples:

(a) Evocation rule:

    IF: KNOWN DIABETIC
             INSULIN-TREATED
    THEN:
             TO EVOKE: INSULIN CTXT

(b) Therapy decision rule:

    IF: NO COMA
             SIGNIFICANT EXCESS WEIGHT
             DIABETEIC ON BIGUANIDES
             GLYCAEMIA ABOUT 2g
             CAUSE OF MINOR IMBALANCE
    THEN:
             TO MAINTAIN BIGUANIDES AT THE SAME DOSAGE
             TO TREAT THE CAUSE OF IMBALANCE

(c) Therapy advice rule:
These rules are triggered in advance if the user requests therapeutic counsel. The state of the patient is taken into account and the choice of drug selected for its expected mode of action, its administration, its indications and contra-indications.

Example:

    IF: KNOWN DIABETIC
             TREATED WITH VERY HIGH INSULIN DOSE
    THEN:
             THERAPEUTIC ADVICE: 'TO THINK OF INSULIN RE-
             SISTANCE THROUGH ASYMPTOMATIC HYPOGLY-
             CAEMIA: — TO REDUCE THE DOSES WHERE INSULIN
             RESISTANCE THROUGH PRODUCTION OF ANTI-
             INSULIN ANTIBODIES: — TO USE MONOTARD
             INSULIN'

The definition of entities like 'Oral anti-diabetics' such as sulph-amides, biguanides, Associated Biguanide and Sulphamide, GLUCO-PHAGE[R], DAONIL[R] define the property links to a therapeutic category and allow sometimes general or, when necessary, more specific pre-scription rules to be written.

4.2.3 Consultation examples

Example 1:

U: 40 year old man
U: Known diabetic
U: Coma
U: Glycaemia: 2.7 mmol
U: Acetest: +++
U: On depot insulin of 40 U daily for 2 years
M: THERAPY:
M: RESUSCITATION BY GLUCOSE INFUSION
M: LOWER INSULIN DOSE

Example 2:

U: Patient seen at consultation
U: 45 year old man
U: Stop
M: DOES IT RELATE TO A KNOWN DIABETIC?
U: Yes
M: IS HYPOGLYCAEMIC TREATMENT IN PROGRESS?
U: Yes
U: Sulphamide fort
M: AT WHAT DOSE CP/day?
U: 2
M: FOR HOW LONG?
U: For 2 years
M: IS HIS WEIGHT KNOWN?
U: Yes
M: WHAT IS HIS WEIGHT (% IDEAL BODY WEIGHT)?
U: 100
M: IS THERE A DISEQUILIBRATION CAUSING THE DIABETES?
U: Yes, minor
M: IN ACUTE PHASE?
U: Yes
M: GLYCAEMIA (mmole/l)?
U: 5.6
M: IS THERE A CONCEPT OF HYPOGLYCAEMIC EPISODES?
U: No
M: HAS AN ACETEST BEEN DONE?
U: Yes
M: RESULT?
U: Negative

M: CONCLUSIONS:
M: NORMAL GLYCOREGULATION
M: WELL EQUILIBRATED DIABETES
M: THERAPY:
M: ORAL ANTI-DIABETIC: MAINTAIN THE SAME
               DOSE
M: TO TREAT THE CAUSE OF THE IMBALANCE

Example 3:

U: Case seen at consultation
U: Aged 39 years
U: Male
U: Obese
U: Stop
M: IS HE A KNOWN DIABETIC?
U: No
M: HAS THE GLYCAEMIA BEEN MEASURED?
U: Yes
M: WHAT IS THE GLUCOSE CONCENTRATION (mmol/l)?
U: 10
M: HAS AN ACETEST BEEN DONE?
U: Yes
M: RESULT?
U: Negative
M: HAS THE PATIENT HAD A GENERAL EXAMINATION?
U: Yes
M: IS THE PATIENT OTHERWISE IN GOOD CONDITION?
U: Yes
.M: CONCLUSIONS:
M: PATIENT NOT TREATED BY HYPOGLYCAEMIC DRUGS
M: GLYCOREGULATION SLIGHTLY PERTURBED
M: DIAGNOSIS:
     INITIAL CHECK-UP NO CONTRA-INDICATION TO
     BIGUANIDES
M: THERAPY:
M: ORAL ANTIDIABETIC BIGUANIDE 1.5 or 2 CP/J
M: TO PRESCRIBE HYPOCALORIC LOW CHO DIET
M: TO MONITOR ITS EFECTIVENESS

Example 4:

U: Age 63 years
U: Glycaemia 8 mmol/l

M: UNDER WHAT PARTICULAR CIRCUMSTANCES WAS THE PATIENT SEEN?

M: COMA, RESUSCITATION, PRE-OP, PREGNANCY?

U: No, consultation

M: UNDERGOING HYPOGLYCAEMIC TREATMENT?

U: Yes

M: INSULIN

U: No

U: Glucophage 2 cp daily for 8 years

M: WHAT WEIGHT (% IDEAL)?

U: 95%

M: IS THERE ANY DESTABILIZING FACTOR?

U: Yes, urinary infection

M: WHAT IS THE ACETEST RESULT?

U: Negative

M: IS THE TREATMENT WELL SUPPORTED CLINICALLY?

U: Yes

M: DOES THE PATIENT PRESENT SEVERE HEPATIC IN-SUFFICIENCY?

U: No

M: HAS THE CREATININE BEEN MEASURED (micromol/l)?

U: Yes, 210

M: CONCLUSIONS:

M: GLYCOREGULATION DISTURBANCE

M: SLIGHTLY DESTABILIZED DIABETES

M: BIGUANIDES CONTRA-INDICATED, POTENTIAL SUL-PHAMIDE THERAPY

M: THERAPY:
      TO STOP THE BIGUANIDE
      TO PRESCRIBE 2 cp OF WEAK SULPHAMIDE DAILY
      NORMOGLUCIDIC DIET

M: TREATMENT OF THE CAUSE OF THE DESTABILIZATION

The expert considers the sulphamide treatment preferable because of the renal involvement. The user may be aware of which medicines are combined in the 'weak sulphamide' category.

4.2.4 Validation

The initial validation data are drawn up in Table 4.2. It goes without saying that the current SPHINX knowledge can and must be improved. It must be capable of giving therapeutic results which are entirely comparable to an expert group.

Table 4.2   The treatment of diabetics: results from 70 cases. The column headed '?' shows the cases in which SPHINX results were inconclusive

EXPERT \\ SPHINX	1	2	3	4	5	6	?
1 : No treatment	3						1
2 : Diet		5	1	1			
3 : Insulin			16		1	2	2
4 : Biguanide		1		19	1		2
5 : Sulphonylurea		1			9		
6 : Biguanide and Sulphonylurea combined						5	

For convenience, only the six main therapies are included in the table but as the examples demonstrate, SPHINX proposes a dose or dose adjustment for each clinical case.

4.3   DISCUSSION

In view of the encouraging results obtained in these two very different applications of therapeutic and diagnostic aid, it is clearly apparent at what point the system expert may bring in either of the two reasoning modes, approximate or categorical, depending on the requirement. The system rates the evocation phase, that is, the approximate reasoning, more or less significant according to the circumstances. In the jaundice application this phase takes account of many clinical signs (which are not always taken into the decision rules) which leads to context evocation and, consequently, confirmation of certain suspicions. Development of a hypothetico-deductive reasoning follows on from this initial hypothesis generation. In the therapeutic application presented the evocation role is certainly less determinant.

Nevertheless, SPHINX allows for a mixed reasoning approach appropriate to each phase and the task to be resolved. Thus it is that in some cases it is possible to introduce data with a strong heuristic capacity into the approximate reasoning phase to limit the research field, data known to be of doubtful reliability or inconsistent, or even sometimes missing data. This duality of categorical and approximate reasoning adapts to the applications, each (being) manifestly important to the medical process.

5

The SPHINX system environment

When an expert system is conceived two developmental problems immediately present: one involves development of knowledge which should come about without difficulty; the second crops up because of problems posed by validation of the knowledge base. It is therefore extremely important to concentrate on a program which, besides an extensive capacity for modifying the data base, provides help to the expert to avoid errors. This second problem may for that matter be considered as an extension of the first; in other words, to enable the storage of expert knowledge as correctly and completely as possible. The sheer mass of data is so great that it is very difficult, even for an expert, to express it completely without errors and contradictions. This is the reason why many systems are committed to programs called 'knowledge supervisors', which look for inconsistencies in the data, detect circular arguments, which put reverse chaining control procedures in check, list all or some of the knowledge according to the user-defined criteria, map out the ways of goal attainment, and which structure and organize in an internal coding a bulk knowledge as Teiresias has done (Davis, 1980a).

When writing rules it is possible to detect four types of error, apart from syntax errors, such as are found in EMYCIN:

1. Conflicts, rules having the same premises which lead to contradictory results.
2. Missing rules, where the system is able to apprehend that in certain situations, it does not know what action to trigger because it does not have the relevant knowledge to confront the situation.
3. Redundancies where the expert has introduced the same rule twice.
4. Subsumptions concern two similar rules of which one has a more restrictive character; for example, $P(x) \rightarrow D$ and $P(a) \rightarrow D$ with $X \subset a$.

The latter two types of error are much less significant in SPHINX than in a system like MYCIN, where the rules are weighted. In fact, if several

SPHINX rules are redundant it does not automatically modify the final result. The system considers the goal achieved as soon as the premises of a rule are satisfied and does not try to trigger other rules giving the same result. In this way redundancies and subsumptions which induce redundances only affect the response time of the system and not the results. For this reason no importance has been attached to detecting these type of problems in the data base.

The first two problems cannot be resolved by programs which use only syntax knowledge in their rules and structure and the elements included in these rules. In fact it is sometimes very difficult to tell whether two rules are contradictory or whether there is a missing rule in a particular situation. Only the expert is in a position to decide in these cases. In this connection a program will shortly be produced which will point out the potential errors in the knowledge base, while leaving the final decision to the expert. This program may be activated through some of the rules, those which comprise the routes to a goal, or through the complete set of rules.

Two programs, COBASE and ARIANE, were developed to form part of the knowledge or to obtain certain information from the base contents.

5.1   THE COBASE PROGRAM

It provides a way of giving the machine a knowledge rule, of suppressing a rule, of listing all or part of the rules base. The user chooses the task he wants to carry out from a list. Rules are entered through a module called MEDIUM which sanctions both a natural expression of the rules with no special coding, and a number of syntax checks.

In particular, the program ensures that the entity is known to the system, and that the values given for its various attributes are plausible. Each time a rule is added, the system assigns it a number and brings the representative internal markers up to date (premises and conclusions). It keeps an up to date list of the goals present in the rules and an associated list of all the rules with a conclusion. In addition, the program identifies and marks the rules premises which are the sub-goals. That gives SPHINX direct knowledge through internal coding that there are existent rules which demonstrate these premises.

Example of rule entry:

COBASE

M : WHICH APPLICATION DO YOU WANT?
U : Diabetes

M : WHAT SET OF RULES DO YOU WANT TO WORK ON?
M : KNOWLEDGE OR EXAMINATION (K/E/*)?
U : K
M : OPTION : TO RE-ENTER THE INITIAL RULES (INITIALIZATION)   (1)
M :   TO ADD THEM   (2)
M :   TO SUPPRESS THEM   (3)
M :   TO LIST THEM   (4)
U : 2
M : HYPOTHESES :
U : Glycaemia greatly increased
U : Acetest negative
U : Stop
M : CONCLUSIONS :
U : Glycoregulation greatly impaired
U : Stop
M : OK?
U : Yes
M : RULE No 14 STORED
M : RULE FOLLOWING?
U : Yes
M : HYPOTHESES :
U : glucose quite raised
U : Acetest negative
U : Stop
M : CONCLUSIONS :
U : Glycoregulation slightly impaired
U : Stop
M : OK?
U : Yes
M : Rule No 15 STORED
M : RULE FOLLOWING?
U : No
M : WHICH SET OF RULES DO YOU WANT TO WORK ON?
M : KNOWLEDGE OR EXAMINATION (K/E/*)?
U : E
M : HYPOTHESES :
U : Glycaemia slightly increased
U : Acetest negative
U : Blood ionograph :
U : pH acidosis of pregnancy
U : Lactacidaemia : hyperlactacidaemia
U : Stop
M : CONCLUSIONS :
U : Emergency biological check-up : lactic acidosis
M : OK?
U : Yes

5.2   THE ARIANE PROGRAM

ARIANE is programmed to list rules in numerical order and to give these rule numbers either at the end, or in the premise part of the rule. The program also provides means for reaching a given goal and detecting circular arguments which are pointed out to the expert, although ARIANE takes no initiative to intervene.

Example:

ARIANE

```
M : WHAT APPLICATION DO YOU WANT?
U : Jaundice
M : DO YOU WISH TO :
M : (1) LIST A RULE ACCORDING TO ITS NUMBER?
M : (2) LOOK FOR RULES COMPRISING DATA ENTITIES IN CONCLUSION?
M : (3) LOOK FOR RULES COMPRISING DATA ENTITIES OF STATE/CONDITION
M : (4) LOOK FOR RULES CONTAINING DATA ENTITIES?
M : (5) DEMONSTRATE GOALS OR SUB-GOALS?
M : ?
U : 1
M : WHICH RULE NUMBER?
U : 45
M : HYPOTHESES
M : HISTORY OF THE ILLNESS CONTEXT : PROGRESSIVE JAUNDICE
M :                                          BLOOD-STAINED STOOLS
M : PRESENT CONTEXT : CONJUGATED BILIRUBIN MAINLY
M :                          ALKALINE PHOSPHATASES INCREASED
M : CONCLUSIONS
M : SUSPECTED CANCER OF THE AMPULLA OF VATER
M : ANOTHER RULE?
U : NO
M : ?
U : 5
M : CONCLUSIONS :
U : Malaria
U : Stop
M :       RUN NUMBER : 1
M : RULE NUMBER → 156
M : RULE NUMBER →  52
M : DO WE CONTINUE (Y/N)
U : Y
M :       RUN NUMBER : 2
M : RULE NUMBER → 156
M : RULE NUMBER →  51
M : DO WE CONTINUE (Y/N)
U : N
```

A teaching aid based on SPHINX has recently been developed. This system has a dual role:

1. First to teach medical students or doctors on continuous training. The system is designed to simulate a consultation by presenting a bird's eye view to the student and guide him through the diagnostic or therapeutic stage. It also sets out to account for or explain the patient's symptomatology by explanatory physiological knowledge represented by the production rules.
2. Secondly, to tackle the general problem of expert systems which were referred to earlier, namely, the pursuit of knowledge base consolidation. Two different approaches are made to the problem of jaundice: the expert knowledge which integrates his experience and savoir-faire; and the knowledge from the physiopathological model. It is considered that the collation of these approaches is a natural way to reveal the deficiences or contradictions of the one compared with the other.

This application will place a whole library of recorded clinical cases at the disposal of SPHINX which might be used to test the system during development. In particular, it would enable the behaviour and performance of a new set of rules to be observed in quite classical situations, and as a genuine trial run.

PART THREE
Validation

6
Validation of the expert systems

Results obtained with the SPHINX system in the study of diabetes and jaundice are presented and attention drawn to the fragmentary nature of these essentially preliminary results. In fact, many methodological problems present when validating this type of system. Merely concordant results between the system and the expert are quite inadequate to appreciate fully the expertise of the system or the benefit it may have for potential users.

Some of the problems involved with evaluation of these systems will be introduced briefly referring to some ideas developed by Fieschi and Joubert (1984).

Besides the validation of the knowledge base which presents real difficulties, many other criteria should be considered when assessing the benefit of an application. The first question (to be asked) concerns the chosen domain. A sound domain requires symbolic reasoning and the use of heuristics, and is not suited to an algorithmic approach. Moreover, the application calls for expert knowledge and experience in the chosen field with the expertise to work on the knowledge base and to ensure the follow-up. Added to this, the problem should have access to data in a sufficiently restricted domain which may be selected without reference to data in other domains so as to have potential use in real-life situations. Potential users should express their need for such a system and it is desirable to consult with them very early in development in order to increase the chances of meeting and satisfying their needs (Gaschnig *et al.*, 1983). Teach and Shortliffe (1981) show that:

1. Depending on their speciality, doctors are more or less persuaded of the benefit of such systems.
2. Young doctors expect more from them than those with ten to twenty years experience.
3. An 'infallible' system is neither feasible nor expected by doctors.
4. They should be devised in a manner that introduces minimum change in current clinical practice.

Firstly, the number of relvant cases found in medical practice should be significant enough to allow convenient development and trial of the system.

One of the main problems of assessing an expert system is definitely the validation of its knowledge base. In medicine particularly, where ethical considerations confine the system distribution to the medical community, this validation is difficult and must rely on faultless methodology. Indeed, if serviceable and usable systems are required it is necessary to make quite sure that a doctor following their advice gives the best possible treatment without putting his patient's life in danger.

At present there are very few systems which have been rigorously validated by well codified and guaranteed methods. Generally, the performance of existing systems is evaluated in special circumstances which introduce biases that distort estimation of their capabilities in actual cases, as well as the expertise level of the knowledge base. These systems are usually assessed from cases which stem from a single hospital department by users who had participated in the elaboration of the system and its knowledge base, using insufficient criteria to ensure their capability. Besides which, validation of the knowledge base constitutes only one aspect of the process: the inference motor, the man-machine interface; the mode of representation and display of data, the quality of explanations produced, intermediary findings which occur in the system reasoning, response time, duration of consultation and the ergonomic aspects (use of graphics or allowing use of the mouse as in ONCOCIN) must all form part of the evaluation. It is difficult to tell at present whether such-and-such an approach to data representation or a particular inference mechanism is more suitable than another to implement a given application. The difference between the kind of knowledge and the possibilities offered by the chosen representation is not always apparent in expert systems applications. The constraints and precision limits employed are not always explicit (Fieschi and Joubert, 1984). Finally, the evaluation criteria are not all of equal weight depending on the exercises, the motivations and assistance required by the various types. Users may be divided into three main groups:

1. The intended user is not an expert in the field and employs the system rapidly to obtain astute advice on a problem that he has difficulty resolving. Example: a general practitioner consults a system for advice on treatment of a diabetic. This type of user takes many decisions devoting a minimum time for each. On that account, certain criteria which are of prime importance for user acceptability must be included in the calculations: facility of access to system advice, its speed of production, its clarity, the form of expression used and the possibilities of dialogue interface.

2. The expert user who is testing the system knowledge and is capable of modifying it and adding to it should the occasion demand. This type of user makes few time-consuming or thought-provoking decisions. The problems of ease and speed of access are less important. Knowledge base control aids are more important here.

3. The user is not an expert and has little knowledge of the domain. This is the case where a sick person uses a system to keep an eye on his condition or where a student uses it for educational purposes. The explanations should then be capable of adaptation to the standard of the questioner. In such cases the importance of the vocabulary and formulation of these questions must be stressed. Few systems today concern themselves with (the) proper interpretation of the non-expert replies and the conditions under which symptoms were observed and noted (basis of all decision-making steps). In particular, where the system allows use of weightings (degrees of certainty, and of credibility) to characterize its responses, there is no affirmation unless the consultant's 'norm' agrees with that of the expert who expressed the credibility factor of the knowledge rules (absence of hepatomegaly does not have the same significance if it is confirmed by a student rather than a gastro-enterologist). Clearly this problem is less acute if the system acquires patient data from an machine and if the system is adapted to minimize human intervention as in a monitoring application such as VM (Fagan *et al.*, 1979) or functional examinations like PUFF where good data reliability may be more easily controlled.

System validation should therefore tackle validation of the data base and the other components of the system: the interface sub-system, the inference sub-system and the sub-system of knowledge production.

6.1   THE INTERFACE SUB-SYSTEM

Two distinct types of system are recognized in which evaluation problems and criteria have different importance:

1. The human operator is directly involved: If this user is not the expert (non-expert consultant or student using the system for education) the vocabulary used and the form in which questions are asked is very important. For example, questions related to the symptoms of an oedema: colour, appearance, localization, pain on palpitation and gradient, involve a long and tedious dialogue for a trained doctor who from his knowledge classifies oedema as inflammatory or non-inflammatory, but are significant when teaching the student how to

look for ankle oedema, in orthostatism, or to improve his symptomatology assisting him to conceive and observe the difference between inflammatory and non-inflammatory oedema, and if one wants a check on the reliability of his replies.
2. The sub-system does not materially involve the human operator. This applies to applications like PUFF or VM which process physiological signals. It is easier to control the reliability of these data which are mainly numerical so their purpose is to reduce human intervention to a minimum and protect the systems with fault-finding or early warning alarm systems.

6.2   THE INFERENCE SUB-SYSTEM

The strategies, aims and concepts operated by the various distinguished systems that have been referred to are different because they were not devised with the same intention. For example, INTERNIST was planned to provide a diagnostic precision aid, while PIP attempts to simulate the conduct of a nephrologist.

6.2.1   The knowledge model

Two models are proposed: the empirical and the causal model. They operate by data representation techniques depending on production rules or as shown in Figure 6.1.

Systems based on the empirical model use a knowledge which does not represent 'in depth' understanding of the domain but rather the heuristics used by experts to symbolize a surface knowledge; on that account, systems based on this model cannot resolve very complex problems and do not produce satisfactory explanations of their advice. This has been demonstrated by Clancey in his study of the MYCIN rules (Clancey, 1983). The causal model expresses a much subtler knowledge offering opportunity for more profitable explanations. Unfortunately, this knowledge is not always available in every application envisaged.

Representation / Model	Rules	Frames
Empirical	MYCIN	INTERNIST
Causal	EXPERT	ABEL

Fig. 6.1

6.2.2   Generation of hypotheses

One of the benefits of an intelligent system is its capacity for developing suitable hypotheses when confronted with a patient problem. Studies of human behaviour show that, in general, the experts generate few apposite hypotheses. Different methods have been proposed to try and resolve the problem. In MYCIN, one cannot strictly speaking talk of hypothesis generation; in fact, the system weighs up all the possible objectives and tests them by a reverse chaining process. This results in a system such as MYCIN may seem restricting compared with method is only contemplated in an exceptionally limited domain. PIP activates its frames through 'trigger' mechanisms and an algorithm, which approximates to the estimation of probabilities to calculate the score which gives the degree of confirmation of a hypothesis on the strength of the presence or absence of various symptoms. If a sign is accounted for by a proven hypothesis, PIP does not exclude it in its search for confirmation of a second hypothesis.

INTERNIST chooses the opposite way: as soon as a hypothesis is explained by a sign, the system considers it no further when confirming another hypothesis. These two opposing methods produce interesting results in their chosen applications, but the methodological problem remains.

6.2.3   Management of data use

The strategies and reasoning processes operated by expert systems may be considered satisfactory throughout the chosen applications. At the same time it is apparent that they do not always agree with the doctor's reasoning, and are often unsatisfactory. For example, the depth of a tree in a system such as MYCIN may seem restricting compared with our own reasoning which dictates that the application domain really ought to be broken down into distinct problems and sub-problems. This is not always so, especially with diagnostic problems where intricate obscure pathologies do not allow independent reasoning of the various diseases presenting.

6.2.4   Weighting of rules and data

Broadly speaking the problem of the weighting of rules is not solved: interactions between the rules are not always easy to anticipate and control. The danger of getting unsatisfactory results which are open to criticism is all the greater since the function used to estimate the score is complex and it is therefore difficult to control the knowledge.

Where results are produced as decisions listed in order of their relative weights, should only the first be considered or could several be equally valid? The current systems have great difficulty in answering this question. The interpretation by a non-expert of the weight difference obtained by the system requires knowledge of inference mechanisms to identify what may be simply an artefact linked to the algorithm used (without actual effect on the decision-making). This makes them quite unacceptable for widespread use. Many should be used only in the last resort. They introduce a total order term to the events which effect decisions, as well as to the decisions themselves; it is well known that frequently this term is not valid. A symbolic interpretation is preferable where requirements can be clearly stated.

6.3   CONTROL OF THE KNOWLEDGE BASE

Current expert systems are essentially constructed from expert knowledge. Development is therefore lengthy, tedious and, more often than not, only tackles a very limited aspect of the pathology. The methods used to develop data bases and the lack of a suitable means for controlling them are such that the manifest of these systems should only be contemplated by one expert alone. In fact, the production by several experts is difficult to imagine given the possible interactions between the rules; besides, systems which have at their disposal means of control of the consistence of the base provided by the expert are rare.

It should be emphasized also that a number of these systems are incapable of explicitly handling meta-data and therefore their performances are limited.

6.4   CONSENSUS, PRECISION OF ADVICE, PERFORMANCE

Besides the methodological problems previously referred to, the difficulty of evaluating expert systems is magnified by the fact that it is difficult to get consensus from among the experts on how to solve a given problem. A doctor does not always, on different occasions, have the same opinion or come up with the same finding when faced with strictly identical cases. As a result, agreement between the system decision and the expert opinion is not a hard and fast criterion nor is it even adequate; it constitutes one parameter giving some idea of the expertise level of the program. The problem defined is therefore what steps should be taken to work out system performance?

For objective evaluation, the advice should be clearly expressed with the same precision achieved by a doctor. Undoubtedly, depending on the degree of precision (for example, the system may advise on patient treatment, a family of drugs, specify the sub-family or specify drug dosage), the agreement shown will vary and have neither the same significance nor the same distribution. This subject will be developed in the following chapters.

7

A crucial problem: validation of the knowledge base

Knowledge bases of current expert systems are established by competent experts. They are not worked out in one go. During system development the expert is led to make numerous changes in the knowledge base, to modify certain rules, to change his mind about the way of expressing some data in the light of results obtained from tests. Most knowledge bases are perfected by testing and correcting the existing base against cases submitted to the system. This process is lengthy and development of the base is difficult even for the more experienced experts. In some cases the expert resorts to programs which help him to refine the knowledge rules; examples of this type of program are referred to by Davis and Teiresias (1980a), Politakis (1984) and Golmard (1984). The SEEK system developed by Politakis provides advice which leads to interactive refinement of the rules. It is founded on a basis of recorded cases whose purpose is to generalize or to specialize certain rules empirically, to obtain better performances. Generalization consists in weakening a rule by suppressing one or more of its conditions. This leads to more frequent release of the rule. Specialization strengthens a rule by adding one or more conditions which make its application less flexible. Golmard offers a development aid for the knowledge base of the SAM system (Gascuel, 1981) by a method of optimization of production rules weightings to cut down the development and test time which is a preliminary to time taken for validation of the rules base. These aids may be valuable but the knowledge base once constituted must be validated.

7.1 METHODS

Besides the 'anecdotal' approach (Weiss and Kulikowski, 1984) two methods of validating a knowledge base are singled out:

1. The empirical approach (possibly based on tapping of cases recorded in a data base).
2. Validation methods which refer to a protocol.

The anecdotal approach is not an acceptable validation method. It corresponds schematically to the following: the system makers describe their experiments and the situations where the system works well. In cases where the system works less well, the knowledge is modified ensuring that the alterations do not create errors for the cases that the system handles well.

The empirical approach is founded on a sample of representative cases that may be stored in the data base. This approach is more relevant. It is used in the validation of INTERNIST. The cases are records published in the *New England Journal of Medicine*. The effect of modifications to the knowledge base is checked periodically against this case file. However, it may be difficult, depending on the applications, to assemble a sufficiently large and representative sample. In addition, it is necessary to provide precise evaluation criteria; the correct solution must be known in each case.

The third and only valuable approach in our opinion, which can be used alone or combined with the empirical one, is inspired by the methodology used in controlled therapeutic trials. It involves production of a protocol with precise conditions of system control, of the cases to be presented (to the system), of the pre-selected assessment criteria and of conditions in which the experts would be led to adjudicate the system advice. This type of methodology restricts bias in the estimation of the quality of advice given by setting out firm conditions for the study in advance. It must be realized that these evaluation biases are significant and that a blind study does not enable the user to distinguish between machine advice and that of an expert; they should be eliminated (Shortliffe, 1981). It is within this framework that the study of validation of the SPHINX knowledge base in the treatment of diabetes is presented in Chapter 8.

7.2 SOME NOTEWORTHY EXAMPLES

7.2.1 Validation of the MYCIN knowledge base (Yu *et al.*, 1979a; 1979b)

MYCIN performance was evaluated in two stages:

1. In a first phase, several prescribers and MYCIN advised on the test cases;
2. In phase two, the consultants assessed each advice without knowing its origin.

The evaluation bears upon ten case histories selected by a doctor unacquainted with the system. These cases were presented to eight doctors: five of them were specialists in infectious diseases and the three others were, respectively, a doctor in training as specialist in infectious diseases, a houseman and a medical student. Ten prescriptions were collected for each case: eight from the practitioners just referred to, one from MYCIN and that given by the doctor treating the patient. The second stage called upon eight specialists in infectious diseases who were each provided with the clinical case notes and the ten prescriptions for each of the ten cases. The evaluators then wrote their own prescriptions and judged blind (without knowing whether the therapeutic advice was from human expert or expert system) the one hundred prescriptions by classifying them on the scale: equal, acceptable alternative, not acceptable. The 800 opinions (100 x 8 evaluators) were tested by analysis of variance to assess differences between MYCIN and the other prescribers. MYCIN agreed the best (65%) with at least one evaluator. In 70% of the cases, MYCIN is judged 'acceptable' by the majority of them. The two experts in infectious diseases are considered similar to MYCIN (62.5% and 60% agreement with at least one assessor). This study caried out by the Stanford group is particularly relevant to methodological schemes, for it is the first study which follows a protocol close to those used in therapeutic trials. In particular, the judgement produced by the system is obtained blind, which reduces its bias. The cases selected were notably difficult ones and, as a result, it was difficult to get agreement between the eight assessors.

7.2.2 Evaluation of the ONCOCIN system (Hickman *et al.*, 1984)

This system developed at Stanford proposes an aid to decision-making in the planning of therapy protocols for certain tyes of cancer. The aim of the system is to make therapy adjustments without moving away from the established protocol, in order to evaluate statistically the results obtained from the different treatments, taking account of the patient's condition. The problems of man-machine communication have been very extensively explored so the system is easy to use; this represents an important consideration in its acceptability by clinicians.

The studies carried out with this system are interesting because they try to evaluate the system according to several criteria and not only on the relevance of the advice produced. So, of 415 chemotherapy prescriptions worked out by ONCOCIN, 189 (46%) are identical (even to the dosage) to the treatments applied to the patients. The authors then went on to draw lots for 70% of the records where there was not agreement. These records were passed to experts for judgement and the following results were obtained:

Classification	Number of examinations	
	Doctors	ONCOCIN
Ideal	68	67
Acceptable	24	26
Sub-optimal	36	29
Unacceptable	9	15

The results show no significant difference between medical prescribers and the system advice.

Study of protocol infringements have revealed respectively 82 and 80% agreement between advice given by the doctors and ONCOCIN with that of the protocol.

The impact of the system on the quality of clinical data has also been analysed (in fact, ONCOCIN is connected to a system which administers the medical records of treated patients). The study demonstrated a significant improvement in the quality of records: physical signs picked up increased from 74% to 91%; information on accidental poisonings from 0% to 45%; and X-ray results from 44 to 73%.

7.2.3   Evaluation of the performance of INTERNIST (Miller *et al.*, 1982)

An evaluation of the system measured against the performance of hospital doctors was carried out on 19 cases taken from the *New England Journal of Medicine*. These were complex cases of patients for whom several diagnoses could be affirmed (43 diagnoses in total). INTERNIST produced 17 correct diagnoses while the doctors totalled 23 and 29 respectively. The number of diagnostic errors rose to 29 for INTERNIST compared with 28 and 21 for the doctors. This study directs one to a subtle analysis of the basic reasons for system errors in diagnosis; some are caused by errors in the knowledge base (incomplete base, incorrect data); others are attributed to the program, such as a fault in the score-computing algorithm or inability to arrive at a decision in the time allotted.

7.3   DIFFICULTIES OF OBJECTIVE VALIDATION

Development of systems-aided decision-making leads invariably to validation studies. These studies have usually affirmed that the systems perform as well as and sometimes better than the experts; unfortunately, they do not offer all the necessary guarantees of objectivity. These safeguards are difficult to achieve because of the lack of a single recognized evaluation standard: the human expert decision remains the reference.

Besides the fact that in many cases the medical problems are complex and there is no single solution, there is much supportive evidence that expert advice is liable to be inconsistent. This variance is the prime type of assessment error which arises from the 'inconsistency' of the assessor. Also, just as it is expedient to check instrument accuracy before taking readings, so would it be advantageous to know the reproducibility of the advice of expert evaluators. These observer errors, that Cohen calls extrinsic uncertainty, represent variations of interpretation between one adjudicator and another, or from one moment to another for the same one. This leads us to conclude the inevitable conclusion that the experts be evaluated before the systems. This is not easy since the assessment refers to a circumstance in which there is not one single correct and final answer but a number of answers which satisfy the various criteria; for example, it is not always necessary in practice to work out an absolutely conclusive diagnosis; a group diagnosis is often sufficient if it allows for complete agreement over or perfectly acceptable therapy. The desired precision level of the assessment should be specified and chosen with care to be relevant to the application, to the decision-makers seeking help from the system and to the assessment options and their outcome.

Investigators in cognitive psychology have identified a great many sources of bias which might hinder decision validation. The experts have to contend with these biases which crop up throughout the decision-making process: from acquisition of the basic data through data treatment to the answers and the form in which they are produced.

In the acquisition and presentation of data there may be a significant order effect (the order in which information is provided is a source of judgement error and the initial data may dominate that which follows); where both quantitatve and qualitative facts are used this may result in concentration on the quantitative data. Added to this are potential errors in clinical data collection: the patient may complain of one thing and the doctor hear something different, a certain dosage is measured with uncalibrated equipment, some paraclinical tests are not reproducible (for example, the determination of glycolysed haemoglobin can vary by 30% in the same patient depending on the laboratory and conditions in which the test is carried out). Further, there is the ambiguity of clinical data and the variations in interpretation to which this ambiguity leads; these data may be intrinsically ambiguous and therefore lend themselves to different interpretations by different observers. In this regard, the study by Bjerregaard *et al.* (1983) is significant. These authors conducted a study which included four surgeons and forty patients to estimate the reliability of medical information in the case history and the facts arising from physical examination; and to find out how unreliable data might allow diagnosis to be made. The forty patients all suffering from acute abdominal pain had been examined by the four surgeons following discussion and mutual agreement on definitions of the various symptoms. The results were tested by a study of variance between the surgeons' observations and the diagnosis reached by them in each case. The reproducibility of the different symptoms is considerably variable. For some symptoms agreement is scarcely greater than if the clinicians had responded at random; for others, agreement is almost absolute (in particular, data on palpitation of the abdomen showed little agreement). It appears also that the surgeons agree more often on diagnosis than on signs and symptoms.

When handling data for decision-making, knowledge of the relations between clinical information and disease presence, as well as the effects of a treatment, is unreliable. For a particular patient the effect of a therapy is equally uncertain. There are numerous biases which occur regularly: 'conservatism' is used by the British to express the difficulty of revising an opinion; the 'inconsistency' referred to earlier which induces different advice on identical cases; the heuristics used to reduce the mental effort, such as the habit of choosing an alternative because it has been satisfactory in the past; the 'justifiability' bias in which a rule is applied if one finds a reason to justify it even if it is not appropriate, and the effect of atypical cases. Finally, the environment in which the decision is taken plays an important part and is susceptible to decision bias; so the decision can be influenced by a majority expert group effecting the judgement of the minority, stress and the manner in which the choice is requested (Hogarth, 1981).

These considerations mainly concerned the problems encountered in prescribing an evaluation reference. Other significant biases in knowledge base validation which should be avoided are the following:

1. Biases linked to the evaluators.
2. Biases linked to the experimental conditions.
3. Biases of sampling choice.

The most significant bias applicable to the expert evaluator is without doubt his participation in framing the knowledge base. Rigorous evaluation calls for an outside opinion; one may not be both judge and jury. Care should be taken to ensure that such advice is given 'blind'; indeed, the assessor should not know whether he is appraising computer advice or that from another doctor. These precautions should avoid conduct which may be either too critical or alternatively too tolerant.

Biases attributed to the experimental conditions are found in practically all known studies. Generally, they develop when case notes are recorded, a condition which does not represent the real situation in which the system is aware of being an integral part and may lead to significant overestimation of the system capabilities.

Sampling biases are equally to be avoided. They can be demonstrated in two ways: the case sample is not adequately representative of the cases that the system has to process or else it tests only part of the knowledge base. The validation sample chosen should therefore be sufficiently large and representative of the types of case that the system has to handle.

Validation studies are generally intended to estimate consensus between system and expert, which is usually expressed as a variance factor. This datum is quite inadequate to reflect the quality of information that may be expected from the system. Studies of variance are just as valuable an index of the quality of both the knowledge base and the clinical consensus of the experts. There is, after all, an advantage in involving the users for whom the system is intended; it allows them to judge its real value.

It has been stressed that the difficulty of evaluating expert systems is sometimes exaggerated because it is hard for the experts themselves to agree. On that account, agreement between system and expert opinion is neither an absolute nor an adequate criterion; it is just one parameter which gives some idea of program performance. When expert and system agree, it may merely correspond to an error of judgement. When the system disagrees with the expert, how often is the expert in error? Finally, it should be pointed out that it is difficult to assess system performance in rare disease cases; the very limited number of such cases introduces evaluation bias into the system.

Many decision-making criteria are subjective; however, even if adjudicators disagree over their assessment method and about signs and results on which their decisions are based it does not imply that they would advocate different treatments or would not report the same diagnosis (Bjerregaard et al., 1983). It is also valuable to work out the range of variation of data input which induces decision change. No doctor responsible for the life and health of his patients can readily accept proposals from a system based largely on the subjective views of other people. If it can be shown that system reasoning is relatively insensitive to variations in subjective interpretation it may be very useful in giving the medical operator some idea of the strength of the system: he may then be encouraged to act on the advice given or else substitute his own judgement. This underlines the benefit of a sensitivity study which should be part of any system assessment.

7.4 COMMENTS ON KNOWLEDGE BASE VALIDATION AND EXPERT CONSENSUS

Development of a knowledge base is a long and tedious process and expert's time is precious and therefore given sparingly; it is asking much to expect more than one expert to set up a system. The sequence of knowledge base development and validation may also be regarded in the following way: an expert writes a rules base for the problem concerned, which is initially assessed in collaboration with other experts to demonstrate which cases profit from consensus and which do not. Refinement of the base may then be considered after examination of the circumstances, where there appears to be disagreement such as; attitudes of different schools of thought and various inadequacies of the base such as missing rules, erroneous rules, sensitivity analysis showing that the system behaviour is specially sensitive to the evaluation of one particular parameter. At this point it may be useful to set up methods to obtain group assessments like the Delphic method, for example (Weinstein and Fineberg, 1980). This technique consists of asking each expert for his assessment of a given parameter and his reasons. The results of this evaluation stage are submitted anonymously to members of the group. If the advice differs, a further evaluation stage is repeated. This process is repeated until the required level of consensus is reached. Theoretically the interactions should lead to consensus by helping to eliminate individual bias (Weinstein and Fineberg, 1980).

By the same token that the development of a knowledge base leads to an introspection which enlightens the attitudes of the expert, and directs him to greater rationalization of his actions within his own experience, it might be supposed that the development of a knowledge base may respond to the following motivation: to seek consensus between several experts who have different dispositions and points of view over a given pathology. The knowledge base is then no longer the expression of the knowledge of a single expert. It targets the consensus attained by an expert group. The development of an expert system then becomes a research method which may prove valuable.

8

Validation of a SPHINX knowledge base: some supplementary elements

This study has been produced from one hundred medical records of various origins (Manuel-Michel, 1985). They were referred to five adjudicators concerned with diabetes therapy: two experts in the domain and three general practitioners who volunteered to take part in the study. Added to these five advisers were a doctor in attendance who had completed the record and given a prescription, and SPHINX. It therefore concerns a study of consensus involving seven hundred prescriptions. As in the evaluation of the MYCIN system, the study is based on a rigorous methodology dependent on a protocol which limits evaluation bias as much as possible. The initial objective was to place SPHINX among practitioners with different levels of expertise; and the second objective was the estimation of the degree of expertise of the system through a discerning study on the consensus and disagreement between the system and the evaluators.

8.1 THE PROTOCOL

8.1.1 The records used

The study comprised one hundred records of known diabetics or patients presenting with diabetes strongly suspected from a family or clinical history. In total, eighty-one patients were confirmed diabetics. The records were from two sources:

1. A medical practice from which only six cases could be considered, other records being incomplete.
2. Two hospital departments of the faculty of medicine in Marseille, concerning patients treated at the surgery or in-patients referred to the hospital by their medical practitioners.

The record selection was not influenced by any test criteria and only complete records were picked out for assessment. Each case was detailed on a card-index.

8.1.2   The evaluators

Three local general practitioners, as well as two experts, volunteered their assistance with the study. It is particularly important to emphasize that none of them participated in the writing of the knowledge base of the SPHINX system. Were it otherwise a significant evaluation bias in favour of the system would have been introduced. The general practitioners, whose experiences vary from a few years to thirty years, have regular contact with the hospital services and participate regularly in post-graduate teaching. They are therefore particularly suitable. The two experts are professors in the faculty of medicine, who provide our reference 'gold standard' of Shortliffe (1981). Besides these five counsellors, treatment was prescribed for each patient by a general practitioner, or by hospital doctors with varying levels of expertise (houseman, head of clinic, diabetologist) and then put in hand.

8.1.3   The study: practical organization

It developed in two successive phases. The initial phase aimed to locate the various prescribers each with respect to others and in comparison to SPHINX. For that, we arranged validation sessions during which each case record was presented to the doctors in identical circumstances. This presentation informed the evaluators of the age and sex of the patient, as well as his weight, height, the duration of diabetes in confirmed cases, the regimen and anti-diabetic therapy if relevant, and the fasting blood-sugar concentration.

For each case record, a doctor was chosen to carry out the consultation, by asking questions leading to better appraisal of the patient's condition (results of further investigations, clinical data, etc.), so as to work out a suitable prescription. This information was given orally and each doctor made personal notes to avoid carelessness. In each case, the questions were arranged in the same order. The one hundred case records were thus examined in the course of six separate sessions separated by two to six weeks. Each session allowed time for examination of ten to twenty-eight records. This procedure was set up to avoid a uniformity of prescriptions which could occur because of the significant number of records studied each session (Manuel-Michel, 1985). Each evaluator writes down on an 'evaluator' sheet the prescription that seems to him the best for the case in hand. This phase was completed by an analysis of agreement of the prescriptions.

The next phase concerns the cases where there was a difference of prescription between SPHINX and the experts. The study was carried out blind. The experts were presented with the clinical cases accompanied with a prescription which could be that of the system or of one of them. They were unaware of the source of the prescription. The case records were regrouped into three categories:

Group 1 concerns the records for which there was identity of prescription between the two experts and difference from SPHINX. Each case was presented along with the SPHINX prescription.

Group 2 comprises the records for which SPHINX was in agreement with one of the experts and in disagreement with the other. We chose by chance an equal number of cases presenting accord between the system and one or the other expert. The two prescriptions were assessed by the experts.

Group 3 includes the records in which there was total disagreement between SPHINX and the experts. These records were presented three times to the expert assessors, along with the different therapeutic advice.

In each of the three groups, the experts gave their judgement on the proposed prescription using a scale of four choices:

1. Therapy equivalent to what they would have prescribed.
2. Therapy acceptable.
3. Therapy insufficient.
4. Therapy unacceptable.

Also, for each case, the experts decided on the type of decision to take, simple or complex.

8.1.4 Analysis of results

The agreement of opinions and consensus were analysed by coefficient of concordance (Cohen, 1960) which is suitable when K assessors classify n subjects in 1 category. It is expressed as follows:

$$K = \frac{P_o - P_c}{1 - P_c}$$

where P_o is the percentage of identical classifications and P_c the theoretical percentage of identical classifications according to the hypothesis of independence of the classification modes. K is a coefficient of agreement which varies between -1 and 1. The bigger the value of K, the greater the agreement (K = 1) represents total agreement. The coefficient equals 0 if the number of agreements equals that expected quite by chance.

8.2   THE RESULTS

A detailed descriptive account of the cases studied is presented in the thesis of C. Manuel Michel (1985). We feel that this sample is sufficiently representative of the non-insular requiring diabetics.

8.2.1   Initial phase: study of prescription identity

In the results presented, the two experts are designated 'E1' and 'E2', the general practitioners 'G1', 'G2' and 'G3', the opinion of the doctor in attendance 'MT', and that of SPHINX 'S'. The results are combined in Table 8.1. It shows the analysis carried out at two levels of precision (of

Table 8.1   Prescriptions of 100 doses

Number of therapentic categories	% in agreement		Value of K		Significance (level reduced)	
	17	8	17	8	17	8
Prescriptons						
S–E2	66	76	0.613	0.711	17.0	15.4
G1–E1	64	71	0.589	0.651	15.9	13.9
G1–G2	56	64	0.504	0.565	14.5	12.5
S–MT	54	64	0.480	0.566	13.6	12.3
G2–E1	57	66	0.517	0.602	13.0	12.4
E1–E2	56	64	0.484	0.554	13.0	12.0
G1–E2	49	57	0.430	0.483	12.9	10.8
MT–E2	50	61	0.438	0.530	12.8	11.8
G3–E2	50	62	0.434	0.540	12.2	11.6
G1–G3	50	60	0.432	0.513	12.2	11.1
S–E1	54	61	0.465	0.527	12.1	11.2
S–G1	49	58	0.425	0.495	12.1	10.7
MT–E1	52	59	0.453	0.507	12.0	10.1
G2–G3	50	60	0.430	0.514	11.8	11.0
S–G3	50	57	0.429	0.480	11.5	10.0
G3–E1	53	60	0.455	0.513	11.4	10.4
G1–MT	44	57	0.376	0.484	11.3	10.8
G2–E2	46	56	0.392	0.472	11.2	10.5
G3–MT	47	57	0.401	0.497	11.2	10.3
G2–MT	45	55	0.382	0.462	11.0	10.2
S–G2	45	57	0.374	0.478	10.3	10.4

opinion): the initial level, which comprises eight categories of therapeutic opinion did not take the recommended dosage into account; the
second level includes seventeen therapy categories and studies the
individual prescriptions including dosage. It is quite evident that the
greater the precision, the higher the risk of divergent opinions. Table 8.1
calls for some critical comment:

1. When passing from a consensus study on seventeen categories to one
   of only eight therapy categories, the percentage of identical prescriptions increases but the result is less significant. This result gives
   substance to the idea expressed earlier.
2. Regarding precision of given opinion, two prescribers may have an
   identical point of view on a larger number of cases than two other
   prescribers, but the result is less significant (compare, for example,
   G3-E1 and MT-E2 for seventeen categories).
3. The percentage of identical opinion between the experts in 56% for
   seventeen therapy categories, when it is 66% between SPHINX and
   expert E2: this latter result is the highest of all. A searching analysis of
   prescription behaviour demonstrates that this difference is explained
   by the fact that expert E2 does not readily withhold hypoglycaemic
   sulphamides from obese patients thereby risking a sharp glycaemia
   increase; and that the expert E1 prescribed mostly the same treatment.

If one compares the agreement of SPHINX with the experts and that
of the general practitioners with the experts, the following results are
obtained:

	Agreement with both experts simultaneously	Agreement with at least one of the experts
SPHINX	47 cases	74 cases
G1	41	68
G2	37	66
G3	40	65
MT	37	63

The SPHINX system agrees most frequently with at least one of the
experts and with both experts together. The result implies that SPHINX
has a high level of expertise between the general practitioners and that
of the experts. Accordingly, it can be of use to the doctors for whom it is
designated.

8.2.2 Second phase: analysis of the different prescriptions

This study concerns fifty-three of the one hundred case histories selected
for this evaluation. In group 1 (agreement between experts and pre-

scription different from SPHINX), nine cases were found. All were submitted to expert assessment using the prescription provided by SPHINX. Group 2 comprised twenty-seven case histories (SPHINX agreement with one expert only). SPHINX agreed with expert E1 on eight cases; the nineteen other cases agreed with E2. We selected sixteen cases from among the records for this phase: the eight cases where E1 and the system prescribed identically, and eight cases (selected at random from among the nineteen) dealt with similarly by SPHINX and expert E2. These sixteen case histories were presented twice to the experts, along with the opinions of the system or that of the expert who disagreed. In group 3 (total disagreement) there were seventeen case histories; eleven of these had been presented three times with the advice to be assessed. For technical reasons, the six other cases were submitted to the experts accompanied only by the SPHINX advice. In total, the experts produced an opinion on eighty suggested therapies which comprised forty-two system opinions and twenty-seven prescriptions from each expert. The results are presented in Table 8.2.

We point out that no counsel from SPHINX received an unfavourable opinion from both experts simultaneously. Moreover, for each case in columns headed 'inadequate' or 'unacceptable', the experts appended the decision 'complex'.

The experts were of the opinion that the system and the second expert were identical (the observed differences were not significant).

Table 8.2a,b Results of the study on non-concordant prescriptions reviewed 'blindly' by the experts (from Manuel-Michel, 1985)

(a)

ORIGIN	EFFECT	OPINION			
		Equivalent	Acceptable	Unsatisfactory	Unacceptable
	80	47	31	2	0
SPHINX	42	24	16	2	0
E2	27	12	15	0	0
E1	27	22	4	1	0

(b)

ORIGIN	EFFECT	OPINION			
		Equivalent	Acceptable	Unsatisfactory	Unacceptable
	80	61	7	7	5
SPHINX	42	34	2	3	3
E2	27	16	4	5	2
E1	27	25	2	0	0

To return to the experts' opinions on the one hundred experimental cases, and merging the estimations 'equal' and 'acceptable', we obtain 94% and 98% respectively for each of the experts.

8.2.3 Estimation of advice as a function of the course on glycaemic balance

We took thirty-four case histories in order to assess the effect of the prescribed treatment with the help of medical advice from further assessment. The treatment administered was that prescribed by the attendant doctor, but it seemed to us profitable, as a guide to analyse the advice produced in terms of the known course of the disease (the only really significant criterion, but difficult to evaluate in a controlled study, given the ethical problem that it poses). We considered there to be four possible development categories:

1. Complete normalization under treatment or steady state in a patient already stabilized (14 significant cases).
2. Partial improvement (13 cases).
3. No improvement (6 cases).
4. Worsening of the patient's state (1 case).

We studied the number of cases in each development category which resulted from a prescription in accord with SPHINX with the different assessors. Results are presented in Table 8.3.

Even though the methodology does not allow conclusions to be taken very far, it can be observed that SPHINX only agrees with one undoubtedly unsuitable treatment twice in the seventeen prescriptions

Table 8.3 Evolution of the patients treated by the doctor in attendance. Agreement of these prescriptions with the system and the doctors taking part in our study

Evolving categories / Prescribers	MT	SPHINX	E1	E2	G1	G2	G3
Completed normalization	14	10	7	8	7	5	5
Incomplete improvement	13	5	7	6	4	4	3
No improvement	6	1	1	2	0	1	0
Worsening	1	1	1	1	1	1	1
Total number of cases	34	17	16	17	12	11	9

advised. This result is of the same order for the experts. Regarding the results relating to the reliability of favourable development, the expert system leads the field (10 opinions out of 17).

8.3   SENSITIVITY STUDY (MANUEL-MICHEL, 1985)

A sensitivity study was undertaken in order to test the vigour of the knowledge and reasoning of SPHINX. It centred on glycaemia as this information was of fundamental importance to the problem with which we were dealing. Moreover, this information was taken account of by the system very early on in the progress of a consultation and it is possible that alteration of interpretation would have had significant impact on the proposed treatment. The study therefore turned on modifications to the limits of interpretation of the glycaemia. An initial modification was to narrow by 10% the limits of the various classes of deviation of the data from normal values. The second modification was carried out in the opposite direction by a 10% separation of the limits for interpreting normal glucose concentration with a similar spread of all other defined classes of deviation, as shown in Figure 8.1.

Level of Glycaemia

Very low	Quite[t] low	Normal	Slightly[t] high	Quite high	High[t]	Very high[t]
⇒	⇒ ⇐ +10% −10%		⇐	⇐	⇐	First change
⇐ ⇐ −10%		⇒ +10%	⇒	⇒	⇒	Second change

Fig. 8.1

The one hundred case histories in the study were referred to SPHINX regarding each of these modifications. Interpretation of the glycaemia was altered in about a quarter of the cases (26 case histories for the first modifications; 24 for the second). Nevertheless, the system only came to a really different conclusion in 7% of the cases with the first modifications and 3% with the second. Moreover, the percentages of agreement with the experts was not significantly altered (they changed from 54% to 53% and 52% with Expert E1 for the two modifications).

To conclude, if interpretation of the glycaemia reading changes abruptly across the limit, the same does not hold good for the therapeutic advice produced by the system, which brings in supplementary data and is not solely linked by this interpretation.

APPENDIX 1

Representation and use of knowledge: symbolic logic

A.1 MEMORANDA OF SYMBOLIC LOGIC

Symbolic logic uses languages whose essential aim is to represent reasoning. This study is approached by recall of propositional logic, which is the simplest symbolic logic and where the idea of interpretation linked to the notion of the value of truth is very readily accessible. The notion of variable is introduced which leads to definition of first order logic and more precisely to presentation of the elements of first order marked logic. For a more detailed study the reader is referred to the following works: Chang and Lee (1973), Schoenfield (1967) and Enderton (1972).

A.1.1 Propositional theory

Propositional logic concerns 'declarative phrases', assertions which may be either *TRUE* or *FALSE*.

A proposition is therefore a declaration, judgement, the expression of an idea.

Examples:

The patient is anaemic
The patient is febrile
The patient presents with jaundice
These declarations are propositions. To each is attributed the capacity to be accepted or refused. They are *a priori TRUE* or *FALSE*.

In the propositional logic language, propositions are represented by the symbols P, Q, R ... which are called atoms.

Examples:

P: the patient is febrile
Q: the patient has jaundice

Starting with a proposition other propositions can be built up using logic connectors leading to forms of words which express more complex facts.

Example:

The patient is febrile AND jaundiced

The connector here is the AND
The phrases so constructed are also either TRUE or FALSE. Five connectors are used:

| for 'no'   (negation)
∧ for 'and'   (conjunction)
∨ for 'or'   (disjunction)
→ for 'If ... then ...'   (implication)
↔ for 'If and only if'   (equivalence logic)

Suppose G is a propositional phrase and $A_1, A_2 ..., A_n$ are the atoms whose occurrence constitutes up G: *interpretation* of G is an assignment of true values to each atom $A_1, A_2 ..., A_n$ of which G is composed.
If there are n atoms in a phrase there are 2^n possible interpretations.

Example: interpretation of logic phrases $P \wedge Q$, $P \vee Q$, $P \rightarrow Q$ each atom should be allocated its 'interpretation': either T or F

P	Q	$P \wedge Q$	$P \vee Q$	$P \rightarrow Q$
T	T	T	T	T
T	F	F	T	F
F	T	F	T	T
F	F	F	F	T

It is convenient to symbolize the allotted true value of each atom P which makes up G and representing the allotted value T (true) by P and the value F (false) by P. All interpretations of the expression may then be displayed as a semantic tree, where each branch starting off from the root of the tree and ending at one of the leaves represents one interpretation of G.

Example: Semantic tree associated with $P \rightarrow Q$

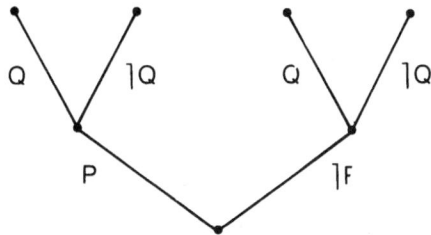

An expression which is false in all its interpretations is an inconsistent expression which is not satisfiable or is even a contradiction.

Example: $P_\wedge\ ]P$ is always false

An expression which is false at all times is marked; the empty propositional expression is not satisfied by any interpretation.

An expression true in all its meanings is a valid expression; it is also called a tautology.

Example: $P_\vee\ ]P$ is always true.

Definition: In the case where F_1, F_2 ..., F_n and G are expressions: G is a logical consequence of the F_i if and only if for all interpretations in which $F_1 F_2 \ldots F_n$ is true G is also true.
The F_i are called axioms of G.

Deduction theorem 1: Given the expressions F_1, F_2, ... F_n the expression G is a logical consequence of F_1, $F_2 \ldots F_n$ if and only if $(F_1 F_2 \ldots F_n) \to G$ is a tautology.

Example: Given the expression $H :: ((P \to Q)_\wedge P) \to Q$
  then:

P	Q	$P \to Q$	$P \to Q_\wedge P$	H
T	T	T	T	T
T	F	F	F	T
F	T	T	F	T
F	F	T	F	T

which represents the facts that Q is a logical consequence of $P \to Q$ and P which is the classic Modus Ponens expressed by:

IF $P \to Q$ is true
  and P   is true
  _____

THEN Q   is true

Deduction theorem 2: (Basis of proof by refutation)
  Given the expressions F_1, F_2, ... F_n, G is a logical
  Consequence of F_1, $F_2 \ldots F_n$ if and only if the expression $F_{1\wedge} F_{2\wedge} \ldots_\wedge F_{n\wedge}$ $]G$ is inconsistent.

Example:

  F_1: $P \to Q$
  F_2: $]Q$
  G: $]P$

shows that G is a logical consequence of F_1 and F_2.
  When applying theorem 2 it is necessary to prove that $F_{1\wedge}F_{2\wedge}G$ is inconsistent.

Suppose $(P \to Q)_\wedge\ ]Q_\wedge\ ](]P)$ is inconsistent
  The expression $P \to R$ is equivalent to $]P_\vee Q$: $(]P_\vee Q)_\wedge]Q_\wedge](]P)$
  $]]P = P$

suppose:

$(]P_\wedge Q)_\wedge]Q_\wedge P$

or:

$(]P_\wedge]Q_\wedge P) \vee (Q_\wedge]Q_\wedge P)$

A.1.2 FIRST ORDER LOGIC

Propositional logic is not capable of representing certain knowledge and expressions of language. Stein and Winter (1974) have demonstrated the limitations of propositional theory to represent medical knowledge such as 'anorexia is a more specific symptom than vomiting'. Whereas propositional logic defines a proposition as an undivided whole, in which it is impossible to consider or interpret relationships between the elements of the field of enquiry, first order logic is defined by a language whose symbols allow construction of expressions, terms and formulae.

The set of symbols as well as parentheses comprise:

T and F (true and false)
Logic connectors $]$, $\wedge$, $\vee$, $\rightarrow$
Quantifying symbols $\forall$ and $\exists$ 'all' and 'some'
Functional symbols which represent functions defined by the elements of field of study. Each functional symbol is given a corresponding integer n which distinguishes its rank and determines the number of its synopses. Functional symbols of 0 rank are constants. Examples of these symbols are:

   $+$ addition and
   $-$ subtraction
   Variables
Relational symbols P, Q which represent relations defined through elements of the field of study. Each symbol has a corresponding integer n denoting its rank. Relational symbols of rank 0 are propositions.

Definitions

* *Terms:*
   Every variable is a term
   Every constant is a term
   If f is a functional symbol of rank n and if t_1, t_2, ... t_n are terms then $f(t_1, \ldots t_n)$ is a term.
* *Atomic and literal formulae*
   If P is a relational symbol of rank n and if t_1, t_2 ... t_n are terms

   then $P(t_1, t_2, \ldots t_n)$ is an atom or atomic expression. A literal is either an atom or the negation of an atom.

Examples:

GRAM (strepto, X) is an atomic expression

GRAM (strepto, POSITIVE) is also an atomic expression

MORE SERIOUS (x, y), atomic expression where MORE SERIOUS is the *predicate* symbol and x and y are the arguments for this predicate (relational symbol). This expression shows that x is more serious than y. The two variables x and y in this case take their values from the disease example.

* *Expressions*:
Atoms are expressions
If G and H are expressions then $\sim$ G, G $\vee$ H, G $\wedge$ H,
G $\rightarrow$ H are expressions
If G is an expression and x a variable not quantified by G,
($\forall$ x) G and ($\exists$ x) G are expressions.

The quantifiers express a property or a relation which applies to all the elements or to certain elements from the field of study. The phrases 'for all' and 'whatever may be' of every day language would be symbolized by $\forall$, whereas 'it exists' or 'there is' would be denoted by $\exists$.

Example:
If one wants to convey that with Jaundice the first complementary test to be done is a measurement of unconjugated bilirubin, one would write:

$$\text{JAUNDICE} \rightarrow (\forall\ x)\ \text{DO BEFORE (BILIRUBIN, } x)$$

Having looked at the component parts of the well-developed expressions of this language the semantics will be tackled as defined by the relationship between the formal language and the particular field of study.

Interpretations of first order expressions

Lyndon's (1964) definition of interpretations is assumed.
    If L is a first order language, an interpretation I of L in domain D (D is not a blank set) is an application which:

  – with all functional f of rank n associated with application I[f] of D" in D
  – with all relational P of rank n associated with application I[P] of D" in T,F
  – with all terms t are associated with I[t] E D
  – with all expressions P associates I[P] E (T, F)

This interpretation verifies the properties:

$I[f(t_1, \ldots, t_n)] = I[f](I[t_1], \ldots, I[t_n])$
$I[P(t_1, \ldots, t_n] = I[P](I[t_1], \ldots, I[t_n])$
$I[T] = T \qquad , I[F] = F$

The same way of defining validity and inconsistency in propositional logic from interpretations may be used in first order.

An expression G is consistent if and only if there exists an interpretation I in which G is valued True. I is called a model of G. For example, one may want to define and affirm DIABETIC (x) where x takes values from the domain defined by the consultant group of a hospital department.

A clause is made up of two sets of atomic expressions such as:

$A_1 \ldots A_m \rightarrow B_1 \ldots B_n$
The set $A_1 \ldots A_m$ constitute the hypotheses of the clause
The set $B_1 \ldots B_n$ is the conclusion of the clause

The blank clause is defined by $m = 0$ and $n = 0$. It is always false because it contains no atom which might be interpreted as TRUE. It is marked as the contradiction: □

All first order expressions may be put into clausal form. An account of the transformation methods will be found in Nilsson (1971) and Kowalski (1979).

A clause $A_1 \ldots A_m \rightarrow B_1 \ldots B_n$ which contains variables $x_1 \ldots x_k$ should be read in the following way:
For all $x_1 \ldots x_k$, IF $A_1 A_2 \ldots A_m$ Then $B_1 B_2 \ldots B_n$

In other words, all variables which occur in a clause are universally quantified.

Types of logic

Until now interpretations have been defined in a single domain (the interpretation domain). At this point it may be observed that the attributes of a predicate or a function are characterized by their order of occurrence and, in addition, this purely syntactical observation may be repeated with a semantic expression. If one writes

GRAM(x, y)

it means that the initial attribute represented by the variable x is a germ belonging to the group streptococcus, staphylococcus, pneumococcus, ..., and that y indicates whether it is gram-negative or gram-positive.

This idea was introduced by certain authors of whom McSkimin and Minter (1977) called this logic 'domain dependent'. For each aspect of a function or relation a sub-set of its field of study is defined.

Example:

Consider the predicate
EVOKE (x, y) which represents sign x evoking the disease y; and given that D(SIGN) and D(DISEASE) are the domains associated with each of these attributes. This evocation relation EVOKE (x, y) may be defined in monotyped logic taking for domain the combination of those preceding:

D = D (SIGN) ∪ D (DISEASE)

and associating with the predicate EVOKE the following constraints:

$$\forall x \, \exists y \, \text{EVOKES}(x, y) \rightarrow \text{SIGN}(x)$$
$$\forall y \, \exists x \, \text{EVOKES}(x, y) \rightarrow \text{DISEASE}(y)$$

Within these constraints, $\text{SIGN}(x)$ and $\text{DISEASE}(y)$ are unary relations whose extensions coincide with $D(\text{SIGN})$ and $D(\text{DISEASE})$ respectively.

Typed language assumes an occupied set of types. Each constant or variable is associated with a type. Each symbol of the predicate P of rank n is associated with a type $T_{i_1}, \ldots, T_{i_n}$ and T_{i_j} may be considered as the type associated with the jth place of P.

The expressions of a typed language are constructed in an analogous way to those of the standard first order logic but the terms must be of the same type as the place that they occupy in functions or relations.

Interpretation of an expression of a typed language referring to n types $T_1 \ldots T_n$ is constituted by:

(a) n occupied sets $D_1, \ldots, D_n$, each associated with a type, i.e. each D_i with T_i.
(b) Assignment of each constant of a given type to an element of the corresponding domain.
(c) Assignment of each functional symbol of type $T_{i_1} \ldots T_{i_{p+1}}$ has a function defined in $D_{i_1} \times D_{i_2} \times \ldots \times D_{i_p}$ to $D_{i_{p+1}}$
(d) Association of each predicate of type $T_{i_1} \ldots T_{i_p}$ of a relation defined by $D_{i_1} \times D_{i_2} \ldots \times D_{i_p}$

In an interpretation the variables therefore take their value from the domain associated with their type.

It must be emphasized that typed logic is no more powerful than first order logic defined within a sole domain. Typed logic makes use of a sub-family of monotyped formulae, a property which was derived from Joubert (1981) and is based on interpretations of a monotyped first order expression and on types logic.

Example:
Given the expression $G = \forall x (P(x) \rightarrow Q(a, x))$ and the field of study $D = \{$cirrhosis ascites, jaundice, hepatitis$\}$

1° from the monotyped logic viewpoint
Let us assign:

a : Cirrhosis
b : Ascites
c : Jaundice
d : Hepatitis
P : IS A RECALL SIGN
Q : IS SHOWN BY

Allocation of values T or F to P and to Q leads to G set of 2^{20} possible interpretations; one of which is represented here:

P(a)	P(b)	P(c)	P(d)
F	T	T	F

For Q one obtains:

Q(a, a)	Q(a, b)	Q(a, c)	Q(a, d)	Q(b, a)	Q(b, b)	Q(b, c)	Q(b, d)
F	T	T	F	F	F	F	F

Q(c, a)	Q(c, b)	Q(c, c)	Q(c, d)	Q(d, a)	Q(d, b)	Q(d, c)	Q(d, d)
F	F	F	F	F	F	T	F

This table shows that only certain combinations establish relations between diseases (Cirrhosis or Hepatitis) and their manifestations (Jaundice or Ascites).

2° from the point of view of types logic
Two types are defined: that of signs (T_1) and of diseases (T_2)

$$T_1 = \{b, c\}$$
$$T_2 = \{a, d\}$$

x will take values in T_1 and the initial conspectus of Q will take values in T_2. An interpretation will thence be obtained for example by proceeding to the following allocations:

P(b)	P(c)
T	T

and for Q:

Q(a, b)	Q(a, c)	Q(a, d)	Q(d, c)
T	T	F	T

The types introduced here are restricted to 2^6 the number of possible interpretations.

Substitution-unification

If a completely quantified category C is satisfied by an interpretation, all clauses obtained by substituting the variables of C by other terms remain satisfied in this interpretation.

Substitution for complete sets (possibly empty) is σ of pairs of the form x_i/t_i:

$\sigma = \{x_1/t_1,\ x_2/t_2,\ \ldots,\ x_n/t_n\}$ such that
1. for all i, x_1 is a variable and t_1 is a term
2. $t_i \neq x_i\ \forall i \in \{1, 2, \ldots, n\}$
3. $x_i \neq x_j\ \forall i, j \in \{1, 2, \ldots, n\}$

If E is an expression and σ a substitution, E σ is defined as the expression obtained by replacing simultaneously each x_i by t_i in E.

If $E' = E\sigma$ then E' is said to be a process of E.

Example:

$$E = \{P(x, y),\ P(f(y), a)\}$$
$$\sigma = \{x/f(a),\ y/a\}$$
$$E' = E\sigma = \{P(f(a)), a\}$$

A process is called terminal if on account of a substitution it contains no variable. In the previous example E' is a terminal process.

Definition

Suppose A is a set of expressions and σ is a substitution one says that σ is a *unifier* of A if and only if Aσ is a singleton. In the case where A accepts a unifier, A is said to be unifiable.

Example:

If one applies the substitution $\sigma = \{x/a, y/f(b)\}$ to
a set of clauses $S = \{P(a, y), P(x, f(b))\}$,
S is reduced to the singleton $\{P(a, f(b))\}$; it is
unifiable and σ is a unifier of S.

APPENDIX 2

Representation and use of knowledge: fuzzy sets and fuzzy logic

Logic models in general provide an idealized representation of knowledge which makes them sometimes unsuited to model some of our reasoning. For example, in a given situation, the context is first evaluated before any action is undertaken. This evaluation allows development of opinion in relation to the data received and is effected on a finer scale than a simple two-value TRUE or FALSE to take account of imprecise concepts. Several solutions have been proposed: the fuzzy logic of Zadeh (1965) presented below, the certainty factors of Shortliffe and Buchanan (1975), and the plausibilities of Kayser (1979).

B.1 FUZZY SETS

The need to use a finer scale than the two-value one to handle imprecise concepts or concepts where the subjectivity of the observer intervenes, led Zadeh to introduce and define fuzzy sets.

A fuzzy sub-set A of reference E (the study field) is characterized by its membership function μ_A which indicates whether an element e of E belongs more or less to A:

$$\mu_A : E \rightarrow [0.1]$$

μ_A (e) represents the degree of belonging of e to A.

For example, if X and Y are two individuals one may write:

$$\mu_{disease} (X) = 0.9$$
$$\mu_{disease} (Y) = 0.1$$

The patient concept is a fuzzy idea, each patient belonging more or less to the class of pathological cases. Transition between membership and non-membership is not abrupt but gradual; this defines a fuzzy sub-set.

The operations of union, intersection and inclusion from ordinary sets are similarly defined in fuzzy sets.

A fuzzy connection R from a study field E in relation to E' is a fuzzy sub-group of Cartesian product E × E'. It is defined by its membership function μ_R.

$$\mu_R : E \times E' \rightarrow [0.1]$$

B.1.1   Operation on fuzzy sub-sets

Operations between fuzzy sub-sets are expressed by operations on their membership functions.

If A and B are fuzzy sub-sets of reference E and μ_A, μ_B their membership functions the following processes are defined:

Inclusion: the fuzzy sub-set A is included in the fuzzy sub-set B if and only if:
$\forall e \in E, \mu_A(e) < \mu_B(e)$
Inclusion is an order relation.

Intersection: The intersection of two fuzzy sub-sets A and B is defined by the largest fuzzy sub-set contained in A and B and characterized by its membership function $\mu_{A \cap B}$
$\forall e \in E, \mu_{A \cap B}(e) = Min[\mu_A(e), \mu_B(e)]$

Union: The union of two fuzzy sub-sets A and B is the smallest fuzzy subset containing both A and B. Its membership function $\mu_{A \cap B}$ is equal to:
$\forall e \in E, \mu_{A \cup B}(e) = Max[\mu_A(e), \mu_B(e)]$

Pseudo-complementation: A' is the pseudo-complement of A if its membership function μ_A is defined by:
$\forall e \in E, \mu_{A'}(e) = 1 - \mu_A(e)$

B.1.2   Meta-implication

To formalize approximate reasoning ZADEH proposes a fuzzy inference rule that Kaufmann called meta-implication. This rule may be used to interpret the following type of reasoning:

'X is Y'
'X is a neighbour of Z'
'Z is more or less Y'

Meta-implication is explained as follows:

If R is a fuzzy relation defined by the Cartesian product of two fields of study E and E' which interprets the more or less strong connections between E and E' (like 'neighbour' in the example given above) and, if A is a fuzzy sub-set E; the composition of R with A, A o R is a fuzzy sub-set B of E' that is said to be given by meta-involvement and is expressed by:

$$\mu_B(Z) = \mu_{AoR}(Z) = \underset{X}{Sup}[Min(\mu_A(X), \mu_R(X, Z)] \, \forall_Z \in E'$$

B.1.3   Fuzzy propositions, distribution of possibilities

A fuzzy proposition is one that may be written 'X is Y' where X is a variable taking values in E and Y a fuzzy sub-set of E which expresses the compatibility between values of E and the concept Y.

Example: 'The triglycerides are increased'

This assertion is a fuzzy proposition. E is the set of possible triglyceride values and Y is the fuzzy sub-set which represents the information 'increased'.

Zadeh introduced the possibilities distribution which represent and process fuzzy propositions.

Each fuzzy proposition such as 'X is Y' produces a distribution of possibilities Pi_x, values which X can take: X is a variable with values in a field of study E and Y a fuzzy sub-set of E which expresses the compatability between values of E and the concept represented by Y. For each value e of E a corresponding interval (0.1) expresses the possibility that X take the value of e.

The possibilities distribution, Π_x^Y is defined by the fuzzy sub-set Y which represents the possibilities of the variable X to take each of the values e of E. Example (Soula, 1981): Considering variable temperature and the fuzzy proposition that 'the temperature is normal, Π_x^Y may be represented by the following graph:

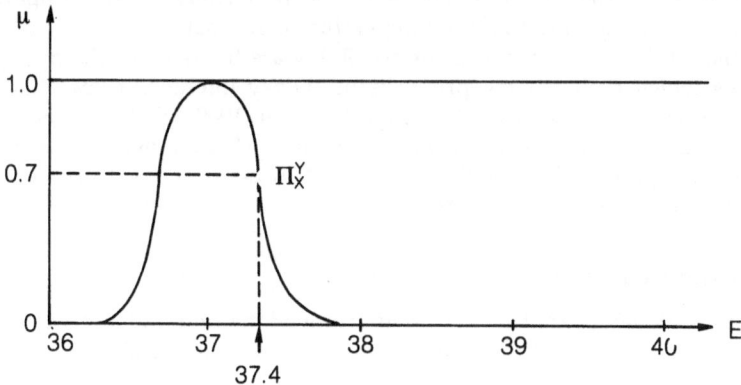

In the case where X = 37.4 for instance:

Possibility (X = 37.4/'normal temperature' = $\mu_{normal}(37.5) = 0.7$

If a fuzzy proposition 'X is Y' is taken as reference proposition in the knowledge, the possibility of having the proposition 'X is Z' is defined by a measure of possibility of Z by reference to Y denoted $\Pi(Z/Y)$ which equals:

$$\Pi(Z/Y) = \sup_{e \in E} (\mu_z(e) \wedge \mu_y(e))$$

The measure of possibility conveys a certain similarity between the two propositions.

Example:
The temperature is normal proposition and its possibility distribution is compared with the proposition 'the temperature is about 38°' whose possibility distribution is presented by the dotted line in the following diagram:

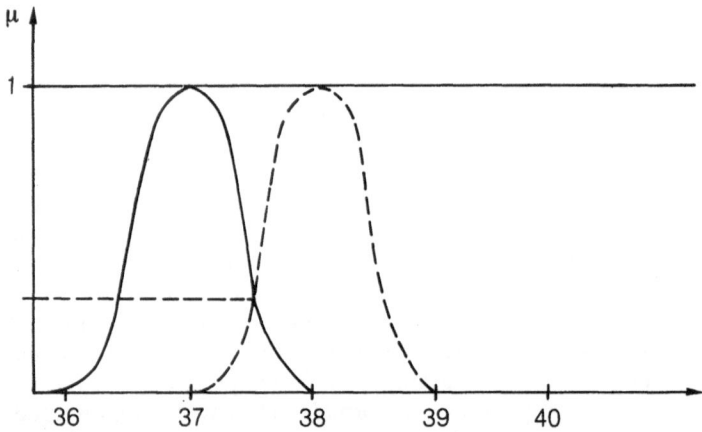

The degree of probability, 0.3, expresses the probability of the temperature being about 38°, knowing that the temperature is normal.

The distributions and measures of possibility are the basis of the operations and rules which define fuzzy propositions. Fuzzy inference rules which are taken from classical and many valued logic (Rescher, 1969) will be discussed next and especially an interesting extension of the Modus Ponens and Modus Tollens in fuzzy logic proposed by Soula. The evocation heuristic used in SPHINX is drawn from these two inference rules.

B.1.4 Fuzzy truth values

The fuzzy truth values are fuzzy sub-sets arranged in numerical intervals of [0.1] in a base logic, L_{4_1} and are therefore defined according to membership function like any other fuzzy set.

If 1 and 0 are taken as truth values in the base logic TRUE and FALSE then fuzzy values of truth TRUE and FALSE may be defined:

$$\mu_{true}(X) = X$$
$$\mu_{false}(X) = 1 - X \qquad \forall x \in [0.1]$$

Accordingly, one may define 'Absolutely true':

$$\mu_{absolutely\ true}(X) = 0 \ \forall x \in [0.1]$$
$$\mu_{absolutely\ true}(X) = 1 \ if \ x = 1$$

or represent 'very true' by the dotted line above.

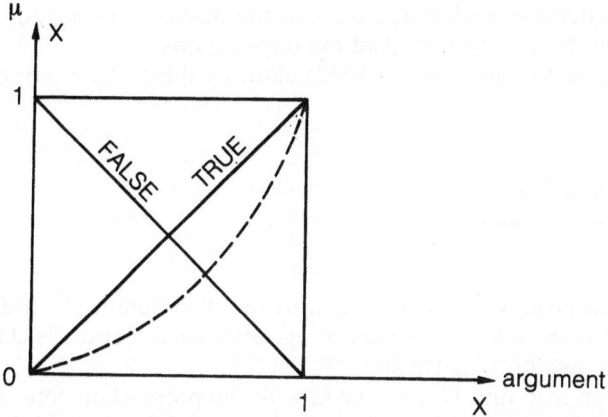

B.1.5   Extended Modus Ponens and Extended Modus Tollens (Soula, 1981)

If P and Q are propositions the *Modus Ponens* is the deduction rule which represents them in classical logic:

$$\frac{\begin{array}{c} P \\ P \to Q \end{array}}{Q}$$

that is, if P can be affirmed and it is true that P involves Q then Q is affirmed. Similarly, the Modus Tollens complies with the classical logic:

$$\frac{\begin{array}{c}]Q \\ P \to Q \end{array}}{]P}$$

that is, if Q can be rejected and it is true that P implicates Q then P can be rejected.

A primary extension of these rules in many-valued logic allows the possible truth values of Q to be determined from values of P (given as /p/), and of $P \to Q$ (as /P → Q/) using the Modus Ponens; likewise, /]P/ may be deduced from truth values /]Q/ and /P → Q/ using the Modus Tollens.

Using Lukasiewics many-valued logic L_{Aleph1}, the truth value of the implication is defined:

$$/P \to Q/ = Min[1 - /P/ + /Q/), 1]$$
$$/P \to Q/ \in [0.1]$$

Soula's proposed extension of the Modus Ponens assumes that the criterion for comparison of two fuzzy propositions is the measure of possibility which has already been defined; and, that the deduction mechanisms act not on the truth values but on the propositions and the distributions.

The Extended Modus Ponens (EMP) allows a third fuzzy proposition to be deduced:

'X is Y'
'*If* X is Z *then* T is U'

'T is S'

The first proposition is associated with the distribution Π_x^Y and the second which connects the two 'elementary' propositions Z is X and T is U is associated with the two distributions Π_x^Z and Π_T^U.

The problem is to find Π_T^S associated with the proposition conclusion 'T is S' (it is essential that Y and Z be defined in the same field of study E and U and S in E').

The deduction mechanism consists of two phases:

(a) A comparison of the distributions associated with 'X is Y' on the one hand and with 'X is Z' on the other.
(b) an evaluation of Π_T^S.

The 'Comparison' phase is made by the measure of $\Pi(Y/Z)$ which is equal to:

$$\Pi(Y/Z) = \underset{e}{\text{Sup}}\,[\mu_y(e) \wedge \mu Z(e)] \; \forall e \in E$$

This measure of possibility becomes a value of fuzzy truth denoted τ which induces the probability distribution (with respect to 'true') Π_{true}^τ such that:

$$d(\Pi_{true}^\tau, \Pi_{true} \text{ absolutely true}) = 1 - \Pi(Y/Z)$$

where d represents between the two distributions, it will be seen that $\alpha = 1 - \Pi(Y/Z)$. τ is the truth value attached to the proposition:

$$\text{'}\Pi_x^Y \text{ agrees with } \Pi_{X'}^Z\text{'}$$

The following diagram illustrates the comparison in the EMP:

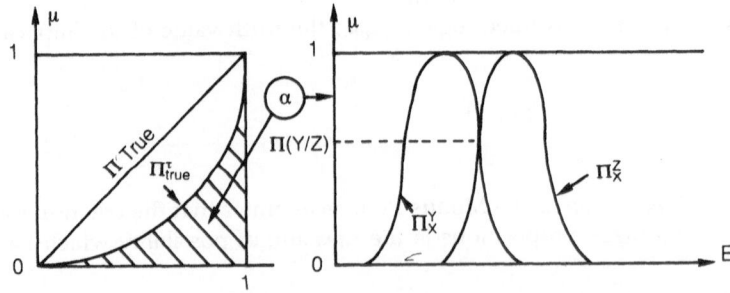

The second phase of evaluation of Π_T^S induced by the proposition 'T is S' defines the fuzzy sub-set S in E':

$$\mu_S(\acute{e})1 = \mu_u(\acute{e}) + \mu_\tau(\mu_u(\acute{e})) \ \forall \acute{e} \in E'$$

where + is the sum limited to 1.
The following diagrams show how Π_T^S is obtained:

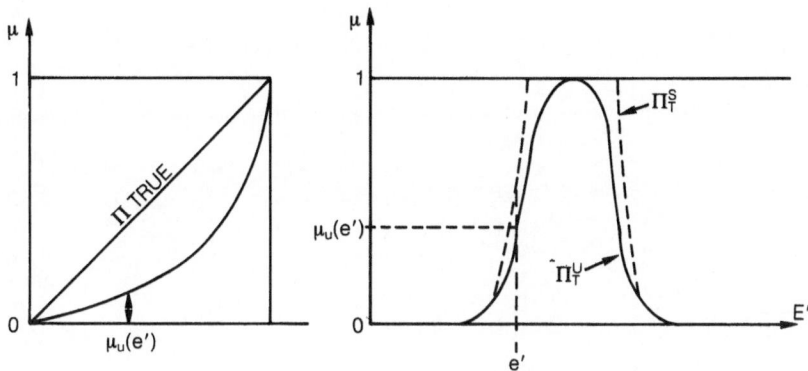

The Extended Modus Tollens (EMT) follows the same two phase deduction mechanism:

(a) A phase of 'comparison' of the distributions.
(b) An evolution phase.

In the following project:

'T is Y'	Π_T^Y
'If X is Z THEN T is U'	(Π_X^Z, Π_T^U)

'X is S' Π_X^S is sought.

The comparison of Π_T^Y with Π_T^U is made in this case not by reference to 'absolutely true' but by referring to 'absolutely false', because it is a question of finding out how much Π_T^Y and Π_T^U differ.
The $\Pi(Y/U)$ is calculated as before

$$\Pi(Y/U) = \underset{\acute{e}}{\text{Sup}}(\mu_y(\acute{e}) \wedge \mu_u(\acute{e})) \forall \acute{e} \in E'$$

knowing that Y and U are two fuzzy sub-sets defined in E' whilst Z and S are sub-sets defined in E. The fuzzy truth value τ produces the distribution, characterized by its distance, β from the distribution, $\Pi_{\text{absolutely false}}$. This distance is denoted β. It is equal to $\Pi(Y/u)$:

$$d\left(\Pi_{false}^{\tau}, \Pi_{false}^{absolutely\ false}\right) = \beta$$

The result of EMT is expressed by M_X^S and the fuzzy proposition 'X is S':

$$\mu_s(e) = \mu_{Z'}(e) + \mu_\tau(\mu_Z(e)) \quad \forall e \in E$$

where Z' represents the complement of Z.

APPENDIX 3

LISP coding of the MYCIN rules

Example of a Rule:

IF: 1) THE PATIENT has acute headaches.
2) The onset of an attack is sudden.
3) The severity of these headaches is greater than 3 on a scale 0 to 4 maximum
THEN: 1) It is possible (0.6) that the meningitis is bacterial in origin.
2) There is a slight chance (0.4) that the meningitis is viral.
3) There is a chance that the patient presents with a haemorrhage in the sub-arachnoid space.

This rule is represented in LISP in the following way (Buchanan and Duda, 1982):

```
PREMISE: ($AND (SAME CNTXT HEADACHE CHRONICITY ACUTE)
CAUSE         (SAME CNTXT ONSET OF HEADACHES SUDDEN)
              (GREATER P* (VALI CNTXT SEVERITY OF HEADACHES 3)))

ACTION: (DO ALL (CONCLUDE CNTXT MENINGITIS BACTERIAL ORIGIN TALLY 600)
EFFECT          (CONCLUDE CNTXT MENINGITIS VIRAL ORIGIN      TALLY 400)
              (CONCLUDE CNTXT SUB-ARACHNOID HARMORRHAGE YES TALLY 600))
```

The variable CNTXT is in this case the context concerning a rule which applies to the patient.

SAME and GREATERP* are predicates used to compare the attributes concerning the patient with the given values.

The variable TALLY refers to credibility coefficients which are given for convenience on a scale from -1000 to $+1000$.

APPENDIX 4

Bayes' theorem and credibility factors

This appendix owes a great deal to the article by Mitsuru Ishizuka and his colleagues (1981) which is the main source of inspiration.

The credibility factors (CF) were introduced into MYCIN to represent the uncertainty inherent in the expert's knowledge rules.

The benefit of using credibility factors turns on two main points:

It is often easier and more appropriate to express the degree of credibility of the rules than the probability in its usual sense.

The function allowing combination of the CF of an hypothesis inferred from a number of rules is of primary importance for preserving the modularity of the knowledge expression.

IF X THEN H C(H/X)	1
IF Y THEN H C(H/Y)	2

C(H/X) and C(H/Y) are the CF of H for rules (1) and (2) if the premises are absolutely true.

Shortliffe (1976) defines the CF through probabilities in the following way:

$$C(H/X) = \begin{cases} 1 \text{ IF } P(H) = 1 \\ \\ \dfrac{P(H/X) - P(H)}{1 - P(H)} \text{ IF } P(H/X) \geq P(H) \\ \\ \dfrac{P(H/X) - P(H)}{P(H)} \text{ IF } P(H/X) < P(H) \\ \\ -1 \text{ IF } P(H) = 0 \end{cases}$$

where $P(H)$ and $P(H/X)$ are the probabilities *a priori* and conditional; they are thus defined as relative increases or relative decreases of the probability of a hypothesis depending on the effect of the premise. This enables experts in particular, as Shortliffe stressed, to quantify the 'force' of their decisions without referring to 'probabilities *a priori*'.

Ishuzuka and his colleagues (1981) have suggested, starting from BAYES theorem, CF combination formulae other than those used in MYCIN and compared the results obtained from each calculation. This process is presented below:

If H and $\bar{H}$ refer to complementary hypotheses then P(H) and P($\bar{H}$) are their *a priori* probabilities.

$$P(\bar{H}) = 1 - p(H)$$

where X and Y represent two observations, one may write:

$$P(\bar{X}/H) = 1 - P(X/H); \quad P(\bar{X}/\bar{H}) = 1 - P(X/\bar{H})$$
$$P(\bar{Y}/H) = 1 - P(Y/H); \quad P(\bar{Y}/\bar{H}) = 1 - P(Y/\bar{H})$$

If it is assumed that X and Y are independent:

$$P(X, Y/H) = P(X/H) \cdot P(Y/H) \tag{3}$$

which expresses the probability of having X and Y if one has H. According to Bayes theorem:

$$P(H/X) = \frac{P(X/H) \cdot P(H)}{P(X/H) \cdot P(H) + P(X/\bar{H} \cdot P(\bar{H}))}$$

$$P(H/Y) = \frac{P(Y/H) \cdot P(H)}{P(Y/H) \cdot P(H) + P(Y/\bar{H} \cdot P(\bar{H})}$$

$$P(H/X, Y) = \frac{P(X, Y/H) \cdot P(H)}{P(X, Y/H) \cdot P(H) + ((X, Y/\bar{H} \cdot P(\bar{H}))}$$

Using relation (3), P(H/X, Y) which signifies the probability of having H if one has X and Y one may also write:

$$P(H/X, Y) = \frac{P(X/H) \cdot P(Y/H) \cdot P(H)}{P(X/H) \cdot P(Y/H) \cdot P(H) + P(X/\bar{H}) \cdot P(Y/\bar{H}) \cdot P(\bar{H})}$$

or:

$$P(H/X, Y) = \frac{P(H/X) \cdot P(H/Y) \cdot P(\bar{H})}{P(H/X) \cdot P(H/Y) \cdot P(\bar{H}) + P(\bar{H}/X) \cdot P(\bar{H}/Y) \cdot P(H)} \tag{4}$$

Consider the case where C(H/X) and C(H/Y) are both positive (in other cases a similar calculation gives formulae of the same kind):

$$C(H/X) = \frac{P(H/X) - P(H)}{1 - P(H)} = \frac{P(H/X) - P(H)}{P(\bar{H})} \Rightarrow P(H/X)$$

$$= P(H) + P(\bar{H})C(H/X)$$

$$C(H/X,\, Y) = \frac{P(H/X,\, Y) - P(H)}{1 - P(H)}$$

$$\text{putting } \alpha = \frac{P(H)}{P(\bar{H})} = \frac{P(H)}{1 - P(H)}$$

using formula (4):

$$C(H/X,\, Y) = \frac{\alpha(C(H/X) + C(H/Y) - (1 - \alpha) \cdot C(H/X) \cdot C(H/Y)}{\alpha + C(H/X) \cdot C(H/Y)}$$

or:

$$C(H/X,\, Y) = C(H/X) + C(H/Y) - C(H/X) \cdot C(H/Y) \cdot A \qquad (5)$$

with $$A = 1 - \frac{1 - (C(H/X) + C(H/Y) - C(H/X) \cdot C(H/Y)}{\alpha + C(H/X) \cdot C(H/Y)}$$

Formula (5) demonstrates the difference between $C(H/X, Y)$ evaluated from BAYES theorem and the MYCIN method; in fact, if α is large the formula derived from BAYES theorem reduces to the MYCIN formula.

The comparative results obtained from the two formulae are presented in the following table (Ishizuka *et al.*, 1981) for the particular case where

$$C(H/X) = C(H/Y) = C$$

The sub-table enclosed in dotted lines (low values of α and of C) gives results appreciably different from those obtained with the MYCIN formula.

	C	0.1	0.5	0.7	0.9
The MYCIN $2C - C^2$ formula		0.19	0.75	0.91	0.99
ISHIZUKIA'S Formula $\dfrac{2\alpha C - (1 - \alpha)C^2}{\alpha + C^2}$	Values for α				
	10	0.191	0.756	0.914	0.991
	5	0.192	0.762	0.918	0.991
	1	0.198	0.8	0.939	0.994
	0.5	0.205	0.833	0.954	0.996
	0.1	0.264	0.928	0.985	0.999
	0.05	0.326	0.958	0.991	0.9994

APPENDIX 5

Other medical systems which employ artificial intelligence methods

Name of System	Applications	References	Knowledge method			
			PR	SN	F	DB
AI/COAG	Haemostasis	[LINDBERG 1981]	X			
ANTICIPATOR	Prescription antibiotic	[KIMURA 1983]	X			X
APES	Dermatology	[HAMMOND 1982]	X			
CADIAG 1	Internal medicine	[ADLASSNIG 1982]	X			X
IRIS	Ophthalmology	[TRIGOBOFF 1977]	X	X	X	
NEPHROS	Renal failure	[ASBELL 1981]		X		
NEUROLOGIST	Localizing neuro logical lesions	[REGGIA 1978]	X			
ONCOCIN	Cancer protocols	[SHORTLIFFE 1981]	X		X	
RADEX	Radiology	[CHANDRASEKARAN 1980]			X	
RX	Rheumatology	[BLUM 1982]	X			X
TOUBIB	General medicine	[ADAM 1983]	X		X	
?	Cancer protocols	[MASAND 1982]		X		
?	Drug interactions	[FUTO 1978]	X			X
?	Cardiovascular disorders	[KAIHARA 1978]	X			

PR: production rules
SN: semantic network
F: frames
DB: coupled to a data base

References

Adam, J.P., Fargues, J. and Pages, J.C. (1983) *BSM Project. The Expert System*, IBM-FRANCE Scientific Centre, Paris.

Adlassnig, K.P., Kolarz, G., Groger, I. and Grabner, G. (1982) CADIAG 1: a Computer Assisted Diagnostic System on the Basis of Symbolic Logic and its Application in Internal Medicine, in *Medical Informatics Europe 82*, (eds D.A.B. Lindberg and W. Reichertz), Springer Verlag.

Aikins, J.S. (1980) *Prototypes and Production Rules: a Knowledge Representation for Computer Consultations*, Stanford Heuristic Project. Memo HPP-80-17. Department of Computer Science. Report No. STAN-CS-80-814.

Asbell, I.J. (1981) NEPHROS: a Constraint Representation and Explanation Facility for Renal Physiology. Master of Science Thesis, M.I.T. Department of Computer Science.

Bennett, J.S. and Goldman, D. (1980) *CLOT: a Knowledge-based Consultant for Bleeding disorders*, Computer Science Department, Stanford University. Memo HPP-80-7.

Bjerregaard, B., Brynitz, S., Holst-Christensen, J., Jess, P., Kalaja, Eeva, Lund-Kristensen, J. and Thomsen, C. (1983). The reliability of medical history and physical examination in patients with acute abdominal pain, *Meth. Inform. Med*, **22**, 15–18.

Blum, R.L. (1982) Discovery, Confirmation and Incorporation of Causal Relationships from a Large Time-oriented Clinical Data Base: the RX Project, *Comp. Biomed. Res*, **15**, 164–187.

Bobrow, D.G. (1968) Natural Language Input for a Computer Problem-Solving System, in *Semantic Information Processing*, (ed. M. Minsky), M.I.T. Press, Cambridge, pp. 146–226.

Bonnet, A., Cordier, M.O. and Kayser, D. (1981) *An ICAI System for Teaching Derivatives in Mathematics*, WCEE 81, Lausanne.

Bordage, G. (1980) *Cognitive Representation of Medical Knowledge Categories and Prototypes*, Communication AAMC RIME Washington D.C.

Bruchet, P. (1983) Utilisation d'un Systeme Expert dans l'Aide au Diagnostic des Syndromes Icteriques, Doctoral Thesis in Medicine. Faculty of Medicine Marseille.

Buchanan, B.G. (1981) *Research on Expert Systems*, Heuristic Programming Project. Report No. HPP 81-1. Computer Science Department, Stanford University.

Buchanan, B.G. and Duda, R.O. (1982) *Principles of Rule Based Expert Systems*, HPP Report No. HPP-82-14. Computer Science Department, Stanford University.

Buchanan, B.G. and Feigenbaum, E.A. (1978) Dendral and Meta-Dendral: Their Applications Dimension. *Artificial Intelligence*, **11**, 5–24.

Cayrol, M., Farreny, H. and Prade, H. (1980) *Fuzzy Reasoning Based on Multivalent Logics in the Framework of Production-rules Systems*. 10th Int. Symp. Multivalent Logic. Evanston, Illinois.

Chandrasekaran, B., Mittal, S. and Smith, J.N. (1980) RADEX. Towards a Computer-based Radiology Consultant, in *Pattern Recognition in Practice*, (eds Gelsema and Kanal), North-Holland, Amsterdam, pp. 463–474.

Chang, C.L. and Lee, R.C.T. (1973) *Symbolic Logic and Mechanical Theorem Proving*, Academic Press, London.

Clancey, W.J. (1979) Tutoring rules for guiding a case method dialogue, *Internat. J. Man Machine Studies*, **11**, 25–49.

Clancey, W.J. (1983) The epistemology of a rule-based expert system: a framework for explanation, *Artificial Intelligence*, **20**, 215–251.

Clancey, W.J. and Letsinger, R. (1981) *NEOMYCIN: Reconfiguring a Rule-based Expert System for Application to Teaching*. Proc. Seventh IJCAI, pp. 829–836.

Cohen, J. (1960) A coefficient of agreement for nominal scales, *Educational and Psychological Measurement*, **20**, 37–46.

Davis, R. (1980a) Meta-rules: reasoning about control, *Artificial Intelligence*, **15**, 179–222.

Davis, R. (1980b) Content reference: reasoning about rules, *Artificial Intelligence*, **15**, 223–239.

Davis, R. and King, J. (1977) An Overview of Production Systems, in *Machine Intelligence 8*, (eds E.W. Elcock and D. Michie), Wiley, New York, pp. 300–332.

de Dombal, F.T., Leaper, D.J., Staniland, J.R., McCann, A.P. and Horrocks, J.C. (1972) Computer-aided diagnosis of abdominal pain, *Brit. Med. J.*, **2**, 9–13.

Duda, R.O., Hart, P.E., Nilsson, N.J. and Sutherland, G.L. (1977) 'Semantic Network Representations in Rule-Based Inference Systems', Artificial Intelligence Center. Technical Note 136. SRI Project 5821. Stanford.

Elstein, A.S., Shulman, L.S. and Sprafka, S.A. (1979) *Medical Problem Solving. An Analysis of Clinical Reasoning*, Harvard University Press, Cambridge, Mass.

Enderton, H.B. (1972) *A Mathematical Introduction to Logic*, Academic Press, New York.

Fagan, L.M., Shortliffe, E.H. and Buchanan, B.G. (1979) *Computer-based Medical Decision Making: from MYCIN to VM*, Stanford Heuristic Programme Project, HPP 79-18.

Fieschi, M. (1981) Aide à la Decision en Médecine: le Système SPHINX. Application au Diagnostic d'une Douleur Epigastrique, Doctoral Thesis in Medicine, Marseille.

Fieschi, M., Joubert, M., Fieschi, D. and Roux, M. (1982) SPHINX: a System for Computer Diagnosis, *Meth. Inf. Med.*, **21**, 143–148.

Fieschi, M. and Joubert, M. (1984) Quelques reflexions sur l'evaluation des systèmes expert en médecine, *Journées Informatique Medicale*, AIM-IIRIAM, Marseille.

Futo, I., Szeredi, P. and Darvas, F. (1978) Some implemented and planned PROLOG applications, in *Logic and Databases*, (eds H. Gallaire and J. Minker), pp. 347–376.

Gaschnig, J., Klahr, P., Pople, H., Shortliffe, E. and Terry, A. (1983) Evaluation of expert systems: issues and case studies, in *Building Expert Systems*, (F. Hayes-Roth, D.A. Waterman and D.B. Lenat), Addison-Wesley, Reading, Massachusetts.

Gascuel, O. (1981) SAM: un Système Expert dans le Domaine Medical. Thèse de 3é Cycle. *University of Paris VI*.

Goldberger, H.A. (1982) DAISY: a Model of Temporal Reasoning in Medicine, Proposal for PhD Thesis Artificial Intelligence Laboratory, M.I.T.

Golmard, J.L. (1984) Une nouvelle approche d'aide à la mise au point d'un système expert. Application au diagnostic des urgences abdominales, Memoire D.E.R.B.H., Univ. PARIS VI.

Gorry, G.A. (1973) Computer-assisted clinical decision-making, Meth. Inform. Med., 12, 45–51.

Gorry, G.A. and Barnett, G. (1968) Sequential diagnosis by computer, JAMA, 205, 141–146.

Hammond, P. (1982) APES: a Detailed Description, Research Report 82/10, Department of Computing, Imperial College, London.

Hayes, P. (1981) The logic of frames, in Readings in Artificial Intelligence, (eds B.L. Webber and N.J. Nilsson), Tioga Publishing Company, Palo Alto, pp. 451–458.

Hayes-Roth, F., Waterman, D.A. and Lenat, D.B. (1978) Principles of pattern-directed inference systems, in Pattern-Directed Inference Systems, (eds D.A. Waterman and F. Hayes-Roth), Academic Press, New York.

Heiser, J.F. and Brooks, R.E. (1978) Design Considerations for a Clinical Psychopharmacology Advisor, Proc. 2nd Annual Symposium Computer Applications in Medical Care, pp. 278–285.

Hendrix, G.G. (1978) Encoding Knowledge in Partitional Networks, Technical Note 164, SRI Project 5844, SRI International — Stanford, CA.

Hickman D.H., Shortliffe, E.H., Bischoff, M.B., Scott, A.C. and Jacobs, C.D. (1984) Evaluation of the ONCOCIN System, Memo HPP 84-9 Stanford University.

Hogarth, R.H. (1981) Judgement and Choice. The Psychology of Decision, Wiley, New York.

Ishizuka, M., F., K.S. and Y., J.T.P. (1981) A Theoretical Treatment of Certainty Factor in Production Systems. Structural Eng. Report, Purdue Univ., CE-STR-81-6.

Joubert, M. (1981) 'Etude et réalisation d'un programme de dialogue homme-machine d'aide a la décision en médecine'. These Doctorat Biologie Humaine, Marseille.

Joubert, M., Fieschi, M., Fieschi, D. and Roux M. (1982a) Knowledge representation and utilisation in a man-machine dialogue with a medical decision and system, Meth. Inform. Med., 21, 59–64.

Joubert, M., Fieschi, M., Fieschi, D. and Roux, M. (1982b) Medical Decision Aid: Logic Bases of the System SPHINX, Proc. 1st Int. Logic Programming Conf. Luminy, Marseille.

Kaihara, S., Koyama, T., Minamikawa, T. and Yasaka, T. (1978) A Rule-based Physicians Consultation System for Cardiovascular Diseases. Proc. Int. Conf. on Cybernetics and Society, pp. 85–88.

Kassirer, J.P. and Gorry, A. (1978) Clinical problem solving: A behaviourial analysis. Ann. Int. Med., 89, 245–255.

Kaufmann, A. (1975) Introduction à la Théorie des Sous-Ensembles Flous. Application à la Linguistique, à la Logique, à la Semantique, Masson, Paris.

Kayser, D. (1979) Vers une Modelisation du Raisonnement Approximatif, Rapport de Recherche No. 49 LRI. Universite Paris-Sud, ORSAY.

Kimura, M., Shimiru, K., Kuwahara, S., Kaihara, S., Koyama, T., Tsuchiya, F., Harada, T. and Yokaichiya, T. (1983) in Knowledge Based Antibiotic Medication Counselling System: ANTICIPATOR and its Implementation by PROLOG, (eds J.J. Van Bemmel, M.J. Ball, and O. Wigertz), MEDINFO 83, North Holland,

Amsterdam, pp. 589–592.

Kowalski, R. (1977) *General Laws in Data Prescription*, Workshop on Logic and Data Bases CERT-DERI, Toulouse (FRANCE).

Kowalski, R. (1979) *Logic for Problem Solving*, North-Holland, Amsterdam.

Kulikowski, C. and Ostroff, J.H. (1980) *Constructing an Expert Knowledge base for Thyroid Consultation using General A.I. Techniques*, in Proc. 4th Ann Symposium Comp Appl in Med Care Institute of Electrical and Electronics Engineers, New York.

Kulikowski, C.A. and Weiss, S.M. (1982) Representation of Expert Knowledge for Consultation: the CASNET and Expert Projects, in *Artificial Intelligence in Medicine*, (ed. P. Szolovits), Westview, Colorado, pp. 21–55.

Kulikowski, C., Weiss, S. and Galen, R. (1981) Computerized diagnosis in the lab, *Medical Laboratory Observer*, pp. 41–57.

Kunz, J., Fallat, R., McClung, D., Osborn, J., Votteri, B., Nii, H., Aikins, J., Fagan, L. and Feigenbaum, E. (1978) *A Physiological Rule Based System for Interpreting Pulmonary Function Test Results*, HPP-78-19 (Working Paper) Heuristic Programming Project, Department of Computer Science, Stanford University.

Laurière, J.L. (1982) *Représentation et Utilisation des Connaissances. Première Partie: Les Systèmes Experts*, Technique et Science Informatique. RAIRO Vol. 1 No. 1.

Lindberg, D.A.B., Gaston, L.W., Kingsland, L.C. and Vanker, D.A. (1981) *AI/COAG, A Knowledge-based System for Consultation about Human Haemostasis Disorders: Progress Report*, Proc. 5th Annual Symposium Comput. Applications in Medical Care, pp. 253–257.

Lindberg, D.A.B., Sharp, G.C., Kingsland, G., Weiss, S.M., Hayes, S.P., Ueno, H. and Hazelwood, S.E. (1980) Computer based rheumatology consultant, in *MEDINFO 80*, (eds D.A.B. Lindberg and S. Kaihara), North-Holland, Amsterdam.

Lyndon R.C. (1964) *Notes on Logic*, Van Nostrand Reinhold, New York.

Manuel-Michel, C. (1985) Validation du Système Expert SPHINX dans son application à la Thérapeutique du Diabète: Étude sur 100 dossiers, Doctoral Thesis in Medicine, Faculty of Medicine, Marseille.

McCarthy, J. (1981) Circumscription — A form of non-monotonic reasoning, in *Readings in Artificial Intelligence*, (eds B.L. Webber and N.J. Nilsson), Tioga Publishing Company, pp. 466–472.

McSkimin, J.R. and Minker, J. (1977) A Predicate Calculus Based Semantic Network for Question Answering System, Journées CERT-DERI. Logique et Bases de Données — Toulouse.

Masand, B.M. (1982) 'A Cancer Procotol Writer's Assistant, Master of Science, Thesis M.I.T.

Miller, P.L. (1983) Medical Plan Analysis by Computer, in *MEDINFO 83*, (eds J.J. Van Bemmel, M.J. Ball and O. Wigertz), North-Holland, Amsterdam.

Miller, R.A., Pople, H.E. Jr. and Myers, J.D. (1982) Internist I, an experimental computer-based diagnostic consultant for general internal medicine, *N. England J. Med.*, **307**, 468–476.

Minsky, M. (1975) A Framework for Representing Knowledge, in *The Psychology of Computer Vision*, (ed. P.H. WINSTON), McGraw-Hill, New York, pp. 211–277.

Mittal, S. and Chandrasekaran, B. (1980) Conceptual representation of patient data bases, *J. Med. Systems*, **4**, 169–185.

Mizumoto, M., Fyjanu, S. and Tanaka, K. (1979) Some Methods of Fuzzy Reasoning, in *Advances in Fuzzy Set Theory and Applications*, (eds Gupta,

Ragade and Yager), North-Holland, Amsterdam, pp. 117–136.

Newell, A. and Simon, H.A. (1972) *Human Problem Solving*, Prentice-Hall, Englewood Cliffs, N.J.

Nilsson, N. (1971) *Problem Solving Methods in Artificial Intelligence*, McGraw-Hill, New York.

Patil, R.S. (1981) Causal Representation of Patient Illness for Elecctrolyte and Acid-Base Diagnosis, Ph.D. Thesis M.I.T. Laboratory of Computer Science. Cambridge, Mass.

Pauker, S.G. and Szolovits, P. (1977) Analyzing and Simulating Taking the History of the Present Illness: Context Formation, in *Computational Linguistics in Medicine*, (eds Schneider and Sagwall-Hein), North-Holland, Amsterdam.

Pauker, S.G., Gorry, G.A., Kassirer, J.P. and Schwartz, W.B. (1976) Towards the simulation of clinical cognition. Taking a present illness by computer, *Am. J. Med.*, **60**, 981–996.

Pinson, S. (1981) Representation des connaissances dans les systèmes experts, *RAIRO Informatique*, **15**, 343–367.

Politakis, P. and Weiss, S.M. (1984) Using empirical analysis to refine expert system knowledge bases, *Artificial Intelligence*, **22**, 23–48.

Pople, H.E. Jr. (1982) Heuristic Methods for Imposing Structure on Ill Structured Problems: the Structuring of Medical Diagnostics, in *Artificial Intelligence in Medicine*, (ed. P. Szolovits), Westview, Colorado, pp. 119–190.

Pople, H.A. Jr., Myers, J.D. and Miller, R.A. (1975) *DIALOG: A Model of Diagnosis Logic for Internal Medicine*, Proceedings of 4th I.J.C.A.I., MIT Artificial Intelligence Lab., Cambridge, Massachusetts.

Post, E.L. (1943) Formal reductions of the general combinational decision problem. American J. of Mathematics, **65**, 197–268.

Quillian, M.R. (1968) Semantic Memory, in *Semantic Information Processing*, (ed. M. Minsky), MIT Press.

Reggia, J.A. (1978) *A Production Rule System for Neurological Localization*, Proc. 2nd Annual Symposium Comput. Appl. in Medical Care, pp. 254–260.

Rescher, N. (1969) *Many Valued Logic*, McGraw-Hill, New York.

Roberts, R.G. and Goldstein, I.P. (1977) *The FRL Manual*, M.I.T.A.I. Memo 409.

Salamon, R. (1976) Aide à la Decision et Enseignement Medical a propos d'une Experience en Neurologie. *Thèse d'Etat de Biologie Humaine*, University of Paris VI.

Sanchez, E. (1979) Medical Diagnosis and Composite Fuzzy Relations, in *Advances in Fuzzy Sets Theory and Applications*, (eds Gupta, Ragade and Yager), North-Holland, Amsterdam, pp. 437–444.

Schoenfield, J.R. (1967) *Mathematical Logic*, Addison-Wesley, Reading, Mass.

Shafer, G. (1976) *A Mathematical Theory of Evidence*, Princeton University Press.

Shortliffe, E.H. (1976) *Computer-Based Medical Consultations: MYCIN*, Elsevier, New York.

Shortliffe, E.H. (1981) *Evaluation of Expert Systems*, Technical Report Memo HPP 81-9. Stanford Heuristic Programming Project.

Shortliffe, E.H. and Buchanan, B.G. (1975) A model of inexact reasoning in medicine, *Math Biosci*, **23**, 351–379.

Shortliffe, E.H., Scott, A.C., Bischoff, M.B., Campbell, A.B., Van Melle, W. and Jacobs, C.D. (1981) *ONCOCIN: an Expert Ssytem for Oncology Protocol Management*, Proc. 7th IJCAI, pp. 876–881.

Soula, G. (1981) Aide à la Décision en Logique Floue. Application en Médecine. Thèse Doctorat de Biologie Humaine, Marseille.

Stein, M. and Winter, J. (1974) Theory development in medical decision making,

Int. J. Biomed. Comput., **5**, 147–159.

Swartout, W.R. (1983) 'XPLAIN: a system for creating and explaining expert consulting programs', *Artificial Intelligence*, **21**, 285–325.

Szolovits, P. and Long, W.J. (1982) The Development of Clinical Expertise in the Computer, in *Artificial Intelligence in Medicine*, (ed. P. Szolovits), Westview, Boulder, Colorado.

Szolovits, P. and Pauker, S.G. (1978) Categorical and probabilistic reasoning in medical diagnosis, *Artificial Intelligence*, **11**, 115–144.

Teach, R.L. and Shortliffe, E.H. (1981) An Analysis of Physician's Attitudes, *Comp. Biomed. Research*, **14**, 542–558.

Trigoboff, M. and Kulikowski, C.A. (1977) IRIS: a system for the propagation of inferences in a semantic net. *Proc. IJCAI*, **5**, 274–280.

Tsukamoto, Y. (1979) An Approach to Fuzzy Reasoning Method, in *Advances in Fuzzy Set Theory and Applications*, (eds Gupta, Ragade and Yager), North-Holland, Amsterdam, pp. 137–149.

Tversky, A. and Kahneman, D. (1974) Judgment under uncertainty: heuristics and biases, *Science*, **185**, 1124–1131.

Van Melle, W. (1980) *A Domain Independent System that Aids in Constructing Knowledge-Based Consultation Programs*, Stanford Heuristic Programming Project. Memo HPP 80-22.

Wagner, G., Tautu, P. and Wolber, U. (1978) 'Problems of medical diagnosis: A bibliography, *Meth. Inform. Med.*, **17**, 255–274.

Warner, H.R., Rutherford, B.D. and Houtchens, B.A. (1972) A sequential Bayesian approach to history taking and diagnosis, *Comp. Biomed. Res.*, **5**, 256.

Waterman, D.A. and Hayes-Roth, F. (1978) An overview of pattern-directed inference systems, in *Pattern-Directed Inference Systems*, (eds D.A. Waterman and F. Hayes-Roth), Academic Press, New York.

Weinstein, M.C. and Fineberg, H.V. (1980) *Clinical Decision Analysis*, W.B. Saunders Company.

Weiss, S.M. and Kulikowski, C.A. (1984) A Practical Guide to Designing Expert Systems. Rowman and Allanheld. Totawa, New Jersey.

Weiss, S.M., Kulikowski, C.A. and Safir, A. (1978a) Glaucoma consultation by computer, *Comput. Biol. Med.*, **8**, 25–40.

Weiss, S.M., Kulikowski, C.A., Amarel, S. and Safir, A. (1978b) A model-based method for computer-aided medical decision-making, *Artificial Intelligence*, **11**, 145–172.

Williams, B.T. (1982) *Computer Aids to Clinical Decisions*, Vol. I, Chap. 2. CRC Press, Baton Rouge, Florida.

Yu, V.L., Buchanan, V.G. and Shortliffe, E.H. (1979) Evaluating the performance of a computer-based consultant, *Comput. Prog. Biomed.*, **9**, 95–102.

Yu, V.L., Fagan, L.M., Bennett, S.W., Clancey, W.J., Scott, A.C., Hannigan, J., Blum, R.L., Buchanan, B.G. and Cohen, S.N. (1979) Antimicrobial selection by a computer. A blinded evaluation by infectious diseases experts, *JAMA*, **242**, 1279–1282.

Zadeh, L.A. (1965) Fuzzy sets, *Information and Control*, **8**, 338–353.

Zadeh, L.A. (1975) The concept for a linguistic variable and its application to approximate reasoning, *Information Science*, **8**, 199–249.

Zadeh, L.A. (1979) A theory of approximate reasoning (AR), in *Machine Intelligence*, (ed. D. Michie), Elsevier, New York, pp. 149–94.

Index